ATKINS DIETBOOK *For* BEGINNERS AND BEYOND

A healthy collection of 90 low carb recipes to help unveil your path to a healthier living,. This cookbook Contains ingredients, net carb,directions and all Nutritional info.

Sarah Smith Miller

ABOUT THE AUTHOR

Meet Sarah Smith Miller the culinary genius behind the transformative Atkins guide you hold in your hands. As a professional chef with an unyielding passion for crafting sumptuous meals, Sarah has seamlessly woven her culinary expertise into the fabric of the atkins diet, transforming it into a delectable journey toward health and wellness.

Beyond her culinary prowess, Sarah Smith is a devoted mother whose passion for wholesome, satisfying meals stems from a desire to nurture her family and instill in them a love for nourishing, flavorful food. Her dedication to providing her family with meals that are both delicious and health-conscious has been the driving force behind her exploration of the Atkins lifestyle.

Sarah's journey with Atkins began not as a mere diet but as a profound lifestyle shift—one that allowed her to blend her culinary finesse with a deep-rooted commitment to fostering well-being. Her expertise in the kitchen, coupled with her nurturing spirit, has fueled her desire to share her knowledge and experiences through this book .

With Sarah Smith Miller at the helm, this book isn't just a collection of recipes and guidelines; it's a testament to the joy of creating delicious, wholesome meals while prioritizing health and vitality. Her innate ability to infuse passion into every dish leaps from the pages, inspiring readers to embark on their own flavorful journey toward long-lasting wellness.

WELCOME TO ATKINS DIET

The Atkins diet is a low-carb eating plan designed to promote weight loss by limiting carbohydrates while emphasizing protein and fats. It involves several phases, starting with a strict restriction of carbs and gradually reintroducing them. The goal is to shift the body's metabolism from burning carbs to burning stored fat. The diet has evolved over time, with newer versions allowing for more flexibility and a focus on healthier fats and nutrient-dense foods. However, it's essential to consult a healthcare professional before starting any diet,especially one that involves significant changes in macronutrient intake.

THE ATKINS DIET
PRINCIP LES AND
GOALS

Principles

Carbohydrate Restriction: The diet emphasizes reducing carbohydrate intake, particularly refined carbs and sugars. By limiting carbs, the body transitions into a state of ketosis, where it burns fat for fuel instead of carbohydrates.

Emphasis on Protein and Healthy Fats: Atkins encourages the consumption of lean proteins and healthy fats to keep individuals feeling satiated and to provide essential nutrients.

Nutrient-Dense Foods: It promotes the consumption of nutrient-dense, whole foods such as vegetables, nuts, seeds, and certain fruits to ensure an adequate intake of vitamins, minerals, and fiber.

Goals

Weight Loss: The primary goal of the Atkins Diet, particularly in the initial phases, is to promote weight loss through reduced carb intake, burning fat for fuel, and controlling blood sugar levels, which can lead to decreased cravings and better appetite control.

Improved Metabolic Health: By regulating blood sugar levels and reducing insulin resistance, the Atkins Diet aims to improve metabolic health, potentially reducing the risk of type 2 diabetes and metabolic syndrome.

Sustained Energy and Vitality: By providing a steady source of energy from fats instead of fluctuating blood sugar from carbohydrates, the diet aims to offer sustained energy levels throughout the day, promoting vitality and reducing energy crashes.

Lifestyle Change for Long-Term Health: Beyond just weight loss, the Atkins Diet aims to facilitate a lifestyle change, encouraging individuals to adopt healthier eating habits and sustain their results in the long term.

By adhering to these principles and goals, the Atkins Diet seeks to provide a framework for individuals to achieve weight loss, improve overall health, archive weight loss,improve overall health.Any adjustments made to the serving values will only update the ingredients of that recipe and not change the directions.

TABLEOFCONTENT
CHAPTER 1: copywrite/Disclaimer
CHAPTER 2: About the author
CHAPTER 3: welcome to atkins diet
CHAPTER 4: **BREAKFAST RECIPE**

RECIPE 1-PG 15
 1.Keto pepper mint hot chocolate delight
2.Keto creamed spinach gratin
3.Keto mini chocolate chip muffins
4.Low carb cranberry biscuits w[ith orange glaze
5.Eggs with alvocado salsa and turkey bacon
6.Leek quiche

RECIPE 2-PG 22
7.Scrambled eggs and bacon green, bell peppers and tomatoes
8.Vegan keto coconut protein shake
9.Breakfast berry parfait
10.California breakfast burrito
11.Keto sausage egg muffin cups
12.Eggs scrambled with cheddar s
13.Mushroom scramble

RECIPE 3-PG 29
14.Cinnamon crumb coffee cake
15.Almond raspberry smoothie
16.Keto eggs with avocado and tomatoes
17.Keto turkey breakfast meatloaf
18.keto french toast casserole
19.Eggs scrambled with zucchini, cheddar and sour cream
20.Greek easter bread

CHAPTER 5:LOW CARB LUNCH RECIPES

RECIPE 1-PG 37
1.Low carb ranch fries string cheese
2.Vegan keto coconut protein shake
   Carrot nut muffins
3.Keto crockpot Reuben dip
4.Vegan ham cream cheese and dill pickle roll ups
5.Mini Mexican pizza squares

RECIPE 2-PG 41
6.Strawberries and wallnuts
7.Keto buffalo chicken wings pizette
8.Keto eggless tufo salad
9.Chill spiced tortilla wrap
10.Cardamom butter cookies
11.Raspberry soy frappe

CHAPTER 6:DINNER RECIPES   pG 49

1.Keto steaks with green onion and caper sauce
2.Keto chili-beef kebabs
3.Italian chopped salad
4.Turkey tacos
5,Curried fish and red peppers over broccoli
6.Double mushroom soup
7.Roasted vegetable soup
8.Keto smoky tuna tomatoes
9.Keto baked tufo with latin marinade

CHAPTER 7:LOW CARB DESSERTS

RECIPE 1-PG 59
1.keto Chocolate pecan shortbread drops
2.walnut Blondies
3.vanilla mousse with rhubarb sauce
4.strawberry with french cream
5.low carb irish coffee
6.Atkins pie crusts
7.keto coconut thumb print

RECIPE 2-PG 66
8.coconut pie
9.pear tart
10.Bittersweet chocolate brownie drops
11.frozen chocolate fudge tart
12.sweet potatoes-pumpkin puree
13.vanilla coconut ice cream
14.chocolate chip macadamia nut ice   cream
sandwiches

CHAPTER8:SMOOTHIES PG-77

1.Tropical raspberry smoothie
2.Banana coconut rum
3.avocado gazpacho smoothie
4.vegan almond raspberry smoothie
5.raspberry-Teani
6.Atkins Almond pineapple smoothie

CHAPTER 9: APPETIZERS

Appetizer Recipe 1 PG83
1.keto swiss chard with garlic butter
2.Tomato cucumber guacamole
3.kale with pears and onions
4.Ratatouille
5.Broccoli barb parmigiano
6.Tabbouleh salad

Appetizer Recipe 2 PG-89
1.Wild rice, sausage and cherry stuffing
2.keto mushroom salad with walnut and watercress.
3.Atkins corn bread
4.Keto herb-butter blend
5.Keto egg drop soup

CHAPTER 10: VEGETARIAN RECIPES PG-95

1.Vegetarian "Sausage" Sauté with Red Bell Pepper and
Onions Recipe
2.scrambled eggs with goat cheese asparagus.
3.vegetarian Turkey and provolone cheese roll-ups
4.lettuce wrap cheddar vegie burger with
Avocado onion
5.Eggplant Rollatini

LOW CARD VEGAN RECIPES
Vegan Recipe 1 pg-100
1.peanut-Tofu cabbage wrap
2.Vegan Burrito Bowls with Cauliflower Rice
3.Mushroom & Tofu Stir-Fry
4.Thai Coconut Curry Soup
5.Chipotle-Orange Broccoli & Tofu
6.Raw Vegan Zoodles with Romesco 7.Easy Eggplant Stir-Fry

Vegan Recipe 2   PG-108
8.Slow-Cooker Curried Butternut Squash Soup
9.Savory Orange-Roasted Tofu & Asparagus
10.Green Curry Soup
11.Marinated Tofu Salad
12.Winter Salad with Toasted Walnuts
13.Tofu Cucumber Salad with Spicy Peanut Dressing
14.Simple Vegan Pesto Zoodles

REVIEW PG-117
CONCLUSION P9-118

Any adjustments made to the serving values will only update the ingredients of that recipe and not change the directions.

How to Calculate Atkins Net Carbs:

Atkins Net Carbs = Total Carbohydrates – Fiber – Sugar Alcohols/Glycerin (if applicable)

Brief History Of The Atkins Diet

The Atkins diet's brief history and development begin in the 1970s, when Dr. Atkins published "Dr. Atkins' Diet Revolution," which introduced the program. The diet went against conventional nutritional advice by emphasizing high protein, low carbohydrate intake, and unlimited fat consumption.

1980s–1990s: The Atkins Diet became well-liked by people looking for efficient weight loss strategies, despite early controversy and mistrust from the medical profession. The diet gained popularity and more prominence during this time.

2000s: This decade saw changes to the Atkins Diet with the publication of "Dr. Atkins' New Diet Revolution." In place of only total carbohydrate intake, this revised edition introduces the notion of "Net Carbs," which focuses on how carbs affect blood sugar levels.

2010s–Present: The Atkins Diet changed along with studies and our understanding of nutrition. More balanced approaches to fat intake and a focus on whole, nutrient-dense foods were the hallmarks of the newer iterations of the diet. The diet became less about following tight guidelines and more about allowing for personalization and flexibility.

The Atkins Diet has evolved throughout time to take into account new scientific discoveries and changes in public perception of nutrition. Strict carbohydrate restriction gave way to a more nuanced strategy that concentrated on the kind of carbs and other aspects of lifestyle. The objective of the diet did not change: it was to assist people in losing weight, enhancing their metabolic health, and forming long-term healthy eating habits.

Dear,Reader

Greetings from the start of your Atkins adventure! Permit me to provide a few navigational r ecommendations for a more successful and seamless journey through the contents of this book as you set out on this revolutionary road to greater health and vitality.

Start with Understanding: Give the introductory parts a careful read-through. Learn about the stages and guiding principles of the Atkins diet. Gaining insight into the "why" behind every stage and meal decision you make will set you up for success.

Observe the Roadmap: Your roadmap is included in this book. Accept it as your partner and adhere to the suggested actions and guidelines. The phased strategy is meant to be used gradually; hurrying might result in unneeded difficulties.

Meal Planning is Crucial: Make use of the offered recipes and meal plans. Organizing your meals ahead of time can help you stay organized and guarantee that the correct items are always on hand. Try out different dishes to maintain the excitement and enjoyment of your meals.

Patience and consistency are key. Just as Rome wasn't built in a day, your health journey won't finish in a single sitting. Practice self-compassion and perseverance while keeping up your efforts. Over time, little, steady steps result in big improvements.

Pay Attention to Your Body: Everybody has a different path. Observe how your body reacts to various meals and stages. Make the required adjustments to fit your unique demands and tastes.

Celebrate Progress: Regardless of size, recognize and honor each accomplishment. Acknowledging your successes can help you stay motivated and committed to your long-term objectives.

I hope that this Atkins Diet Book for Beginners will help you reach your goals of living a better lifestyle with clarity, self-assurance, and success.

Warm regards,
Sarah Smith Miller

BREAKFAST RECIPE
Recipe 1
Atkins Keto Peppermint Hot Chocolate Delight2.3g
Net Carbs
Prep Time: 5 Minutes

Style:American
Cook Time: 5 Minutes
Phase: Phase 1
Difficulty: Easy
2 SERVINGS
212.4cal
Calories

COMPOSITION
15 fluid ounces Chocolate Delight Atkins Milk tremble
4 tsp heavy cream for whipping
1/8 tspn essence of peppermint
1/4 tsp unsweetened cocoa powder
DIRECTIONS
1.Heat the shake (one full shake plus ½ cup), two tablespoons of cream, and peppermint extract in a medium saucepan over medium heat. Stir often until steaming and bubbles start to form around the rims, about five minutes.
2.Beat the remaining 2 tablespoons heavy cream to soft peaks in a separate bowl.
Pour about a cup of peppermint hot chocolate into each of the two mugs. Add a generous tablespoon of the whipped cream on top, then evenly distribute the chocolate powder. If preferred, garnish with a fresh peppermint leaf. As stated, one cup equals one serving.
COOKING TIP
This simple keto hot cocoa can be adapted with your favorite flavor! Replace the peppermint extract with your favorite flavor extract for an endless variety of warming hot cocoa drinks. The key to this recipe is to keep an eye on it while heating on the stove, stirring frequently to prevent skin from forming and prevent it from coming to a boil or scorching.

Atkins Keto Creamed Spinach Gratin2.7g

Net Carbs

Prep Time: 10 Minutes

Style:French

Cook Time: 50 Minutes

Phase: Phase 2

Difficulty: Moderate

8 SERVINGS *9.8g

Protein

13.5g

Fat

2.2g

Fiber

170.8cal

Calories

COMPOSITION

Fresh baby spinach, 908 grams

One tablespoon unsalted butter

Half a cup of freshly cut scallions, bulb and tips

One teaspoon of raw garlic

Three tsp of cream cheese

Dijon mustard, two tsp

half a teaspoon of ground black pepper

One-fourth cup of heavy cream for whipping

1 cup of unsweetened almond milk

Four ounces of Gruyere

Two teaspoons of extremely finely milled, gluten-free almond flour

One ounce of crushed parmesan cheese

DIRECTIONS

1.Preheat the oven to 400°F. Use one teaspoon of butter to grease a two-quart baking dish.

Place 1 ½ cups water and 1 teaspoon salt in a large stock pot and heat to a simmer. After lowering the heat to medium-low, add the spinach and wait until some of it wilts. Continue adding spinach until it wilts completely, which should take approximately ten minutes. Transfer to a strainer and put aside.

2Heat the remaining tablespoon of butter in the big stock pot over medium heat. Add the scallion and cook for about 3 minutes, or until softened. After adding the garlic, sauté it for a further 30 seconds or until fragrant. Stir in the remaining ½ teaspoon salt, pepper, Dijon mustard, and cream cheese, stirring until the cream cheese is fully melted. After adding the cream and almond milk, whisk over medium heat for an additional three to five minutes, or until simmering and starting to thicken. Take off the heat and mix in 3 ounces (or about ¾ cup) of shredded Gruyere, stirring until it melts.

3.Press as much water out of the spinach as possible with the back of a wooden spoon. Chop coarsely, then add to the pot with the sauce, folding to coat the spinach evenly. Fill baking dish with prepared mixture. Place the remaining grated gruyere cheese on top of the creamed spinach, then equally scatter almond flour over the dish. Finally, sprinkle grated parmesan cheese on top. Bake for 20 to 25 minutes, or until the spinach is bubbling around the edges and the top is golden. To create a lovely, browned parmesan top, broil for a final two to three minutes. While heated, serve.

Atkins Keto Mini Chocolate Chip Muffins 2.7g
Net Carbs
Prep Time: 10 Minutes
Style:American
Cook Time: 15 Minutes
Phase: Phase 2
24 SERVINGS1.7g
Protein
5.2g
Fat
2.1g
Fiber
64.7cal
COMPOSITION
1/3 cup blanched almond flour
Half a cup of sucrose-based sweetener (sugar alternative)
one-third cup coconut flour
One teaspoon of Double Acting Straight Phosphate Baking Powder
1/4 teaspoon salt and 3/4 teaspoon xanthan gum
Half a cup of Cultured Sour Cream

Two tablespoons of stick unsalted butter
Two teaspoons of heavy cream
One fluid ounce of tap water
Two tsp of extract from vanilla beans
4 ounces Sugar-Free Chocolate Chips from Lily
DIRECTIONS
Preheat the oven to 350°F. 24 small muffin wells should be greased or lined with paper liners.
Almond flour, sugar substitute, coconut flour, xanthan gum, baking powder, and salt should all be combined in a bowl.
In a separate bowl, beat the sour cream.

Atkins Low Carb Cranberry Biscuits with Orange Glaze3.1gNet Carbs
Prep Time: 20 Minutes
Style:American
Cook Time: 15 Minutes
Phase: Phase 2
Difficulty: Moderate
12 SERVINGS3.2g
Protein
9.6g
Fat
2.7g
Fiber

119.4cal
Calories
COMPOSITION
2 lbs. of raw egg
Five teaspoons of unsalted butter
Half a cup of extremely finely milled, gluten-free almond flour
Six tsp of coconut flour
Seven tablespoons of sugar-free erythritol-containing powdered monkfruit sweetener, Lakanto

One tablespoon of low-sodium baking powder
One-half tsp xanthan gum
Half a teaspoon of table salt
One-fourth cup flaxseed meal
1/2 cup of unsweetened almond milk
One tablespoon of apple cider vinegar
1 cup of cranberries, frozen
two tsp of juice from fresh oranges
One tablespoon of recently harvested orange peel
DIRECTIONS
1.Let the eggs reach room temperature, then melt the ¼ cup of butter and set aside.
Turn the oven on to 400°F.
Sift almond flour, coconut flour, baking powder, xanthan gum, two teaspoons
powdered sweetener, and salt into a big basin. Add the ground flaxsecan eds and
whisk until well blended.
Whisk the eggs, vinegar, and almond milk in a small bowl.
2.Add the almond milk and melted butter to the big bowl containing the flours.
COOKING ADVICE
Treat this dough gently, and the result will be soft, fluffy biscuits. The leavening
power of baking powder and you apple cider vinegar is what gives these biscuits
their fluff. Overmixing might cause the baking powder to activate too soon, resulting
in dense and flat biscuits. 3.slightly stir until all the flours are slightly moistened,
then fold in the chopped cranberries and delicately spoon the batter onto thie
baking sheet. These will maintain their fluff and crumble with every mouthful if you
handle them with care!

Atkins Eggs with Avocado, Salsa and Turkey Bacon5.7gNet Carbs
Prep Time: 5 Minutes
Style:American
Cook Time: 15 Minutes
Phase: Phase 2
Difficulty: Moderate
 31.3g
Protein
39g
Fat
6.3g
Fiber
515.6cal
Calories

COMPOSITION
Two ounces of cooked Bacon from Turkey
Half of the fruit is seedless and skinless. Avocados from California
One ounce of salsa
Two huge (whole) eggs
DIRECTIONS
Make Salsa Cruda according to the Atkins recipe or use 2
tablespoons of your favorite no-sugar salsa.

Slices of turkey bacon should be cooked until crispy over medium-
high heat in a nonstick skillet.
Cut avocado into slices.
Fry the eggs (or, if preferred, scramble or poach).
Arrange to serve the eggs with sliced avocado, salsa on top, and
turkey bacon on the side.
COOKING ADVICE
Depending on whether you're cooking for one person or a large
group, you may adjust the serving settings above to determine how
much of each ingredient is needed.

Atkins Leek Quiche19.7gNet Carbs
Prep Time: 15 Minutes
Style:Other
Cook Time: 45 Minutes
Phase: Phase 3
6 SERVINGS
22.2g
Protein
35.5g
Fat
3.9g
Fiber
490.2cal
Calories

COMPOSITION
Eight pieces of Atkins Pie Crust
Stick of one tablespoon unsalted butter
One and a half pounds of leeks
Half a cup of heavy cream
Three huge (whole) eggs
Half a teaspoon of salt
1/4 tsp black pepper
one cup of Gruyere cheese, shredded
DIRECTIONS
1.Make one recipe for Atkins Pie Crust. Bake the pie crust in advance according to the recipe. After prebaking the shell, fill it with the filling (follow the directions).

2.Set the oven to 350°F. Melt butter in a medium skillet over medium heat. Add the chopped leeks and cook for 5 to 6 minutes, stirring now and again, until they become tender. Take off the heat and whisk in the cream. Give it five minutes.
3.Meanwhile, mix the eggs with the salt and pepper in a medium-sized basin. Mix the cream and leeks with the egg mixture. Cover the bottom of the pie shell with ¾ cup of cheese.
4.Spoon egg mixture into pie crust that has been prepared beforehand; top with remaining cheese. Bake for 45 minutes, or until the top is golden and the center is just set. If needed, activate the broiler and broil for 6 minutes from element 2, or until the top begins to brown.

Recipe 2

Atkins Scrambled Eggs with Bacon, Green Bell Peppers and Tomato8.3g
Net CarbsPrep Time: 10 Minutes
Style:American
Cook Time: 10 Minutes
Phase: Phase 2
Difficulty: Moderate

1 SERVING24.4g
Protein
22g
Fat
3.5g
Fiber
340.4calories

INGREDIENTS
1 large whole (3" diameter) Red Tomato
2 medium slice (yield after cooking) Bacon
1/2 cup chopped Green Sweet Pepper
2 large Eggs (Whole)
1/8 cup shredded Cheddar Cheese

DIRECTIONS
1.Cut tomato into two or three thick slices, then arrange on a platter.
Add freshly ground black pepper and salt for seasoning; put aside.
2.Cook bacon until it becomes crispy. Using a paper towel, wipe off
any extra oil before applying it to the tomato slices.
3.In the same skillet as the bacon, sauté the diced green bell pepper for
two to three minutes (drain off excess grease first). After lightly
beating the eggs, mix them with the green bell peppers. Cook the eggs
until they solidify.
4.After the tomatoes, arrange the bacon and eggs on top. Top with 2
tablespoons of cheese; melt in the microwave for 30 seconds or under
the broiler for a minute.

Atkins Vegan Keto Coconut Protein Shake1.3g
Net CarbsPrep Time: 5 Minutes
Style:American
Cook Time: 0 Minutes
Phase: Phase 1
Difficulty: Moderate
1 SERVING
24.4g
Protein
5.6g
Fat
1g
Fiber
158.7cal
Calories
COMPOSITION
1 cup of unsweetened coconut milk
One ounce of ProPlus Soy Protein Isolate from Protein Technologies International
One-half tsp vanilla extract
DIRECTIONS
1.For non-vegans or vegetarians, whey protein powder may be used instead; just add 1g NC to the total NC content.
2.In a blender, combine all ingredients and 2-4 ice cubes (depending on desired thickness). Think about substituting or adding coconut extract for the vanilla. Mix well and taste.

Atkins Breakfast Berry Parfait 11.8g
Net Carbs
Prep Time: 15 Minutes
Style:American
Cook Time: 0 Minutes
Phase: Phase 2
Difficulty: Moderate
4 SERVINGS
10.3g
Protein
25.1g
Fat

7.8g
Fiber
337.1cal
Calories

INGREDIENTS
2 cups Raspberries
1 1/2 cup, wholes Strawberries
2 1/2 tablespoons Sucralose Based Sweetener (Sugar Substitute)
1 cup Heavy Cream
1 tablespoon Vanilla Extract
6 ounces Greek Yogurt - Plain (Container)
1 bar Atkins Strawberry Shortcake Bar

Blend 1 1/2 cups each of strawberries and raspberries in a blender with 1 1/2 tablespoons of sugar substitute.
Beat heavy cream, remaining 1 tablespoon sugar substitute, and vanilla in a large mixing bowl on medium speed with an electric mixer until soft peaks form. Beat in 1 1/2 single serving containers of yogurt until stiff peaks form.
Make at least two layers of each of the berry mixture, cream filling, and crumbled Atkins bar in four parfait glasses.
Place a few of the leftover 1/2 cup raspberries on top of each before serving.

California breakfast with burrito
SET UP TIME
Cooking time: 5 minutes; 55 minutes
four large potatoes.
Three teaspoons of olive oil
Two and a half tsp paprika
One tsp of salt with garlic
One tsp of kosher salt
one and a half teaspoons of recently cracked black pepper
680 grams, or 1 1/2 pounds ripe tomatoes, diced to a size of ¼ to ½ inch (6 to 12-mm) dice

Finely dice 1/2 big white onion (¾ cup/95 g).
One or two finely chopped jalapeño peppers (remove the seeds
and membranes for a softer salsa)
20 g or 1/2 cup finely cut cilantro leaves
One tablespoon of freshly squeezed lime juice
The Tortilla
Four bacon slices (or cooked sausage or chorizo)
Eight big eggs
One tablespoon of olive oil or unsalted butter
Four huge wheat tortillas
One cup, or 115 grams Cheddar cheese, grated
One cup, or 165 grams Pico de Gallo
Two cups, or 280 grams Ideal Potatoes for Roasting
Two mature avocados, halved, seeded, and cut
One dash of chipotle salsa
DIRECTIONS:
Prepare the gallo de pico. The tomatoes, onion, jalapeño, cilantro,
and lime juice should all be combined in a big bowl. Toss gently to
mix. Add salt to taste to season.
Preheat the oven to 425°F (220°C) in order to prepare the
potatoes.
Use parchment paper to line a baking sheet.

Transfer the potatoes to the baking sheet that has been ready.
Once the ingredients are properly distributed, toss the potatoes
with the oil, paprika, garlic salt, kosher salt, and pepper.

After placing the baking sheet in the oven, bake it for twenty
minutes. Take out of the oven and use tongs to stir the potatoes.
Return the baking sheet to the oven and continue baking for
twenty more minutes.

 Take off the baking sheet, give the potatoes one more toss, put
them back in the oven, and roast for a further 10 to 15 minutes, or
until they are crispy and golden. Take out of the oven, taste and
adjust the salt, and serve.

The Tortilla
In a large cast-iron pan, cook the bacon over medium-high heat. Once it cools, break it into tiny pieces.
In a bowl, crack the eggs and whisk until smooth.
Heat a large pan over medium heat to melt the butter. Gently scramble the eggs after adding them. Add pepper and salt for seasoning.
To make each tortilla as flexible as possible, warm it over an open flame. As an alternative, if your stove is electric, reheat the tortillas in the microwave in 30-second increments until they are well heated. Lay the tortillas out on a spotless, level surface to assemble. To ensure that every portion of the tortilla is flavorful when rolled up, spread the cooked eggs equally over each one in a line. Next, add the bacon, cheese, pico de gallo, roasted potatoes, and sliced avocado.
Roll up the burritos by tucking in the tortilla ends. Serve right away with the salsa on the side.

Atkins Keto Sausage and Egg Muffin Cups2g
Net Carbs
Prep Time: 10 Minutes
Style:American
Cook Time: 30 Minutes
Phase: Phase 1
Difficulty: Moderate
6 SERVINGS
30.8g
Protein
32.8g
Fat
0.5g
Fiber
436.8cal
Calories

INGREDIENTS
12 ounces Pork Italian Sausage
2/3 pound Ground Turkey
2/3 cup chopped Sweet Red Peppers
13 large Eggs (Whole)
1 tablespoon Parsley (Dried)
1/2 teaspoon Salt

1/4 teaspoon Black Pepper
1/4 teaspoon leaf Dried Thyme Leaves
1/4 teaspoon Paprika
1/8 teaspoon Nutmeg (Ground)
1/8 teaspoon Red or Cayenne Pepper
DIRECTIONS
1.Turn the oven on to 350°F. Muffin tin with twelve wells: grease it.
2.Sausage and ground turkey should be well combined.
Add one egg, diced red bell pepper, parsley, paprika, nutmeg, cayenne, salt, and pepper. Using your hands, combine all the ingredients and mix until well combined.
Evenly distribute the sausage mixture (approximately 66 grams per muffin well) across the 12 muffin wells. Making ensuring there are no holes in the mixture, press the sausage mixture up and slightly over the well rims to form an outer layer.
3.Place one egg into each well and pop them straight into the oven. Bake the eggs for 25 to 30 minutes, or until set. If you choose, top with cheese, salsa, or hot sauce (don't forget to add the extra grams of NC!).
The number of ingredients needed will be displayed when you adjust the serving settings above, regardless of whether you're cooking for a family or just yourself.
28 days back
4.1 piece of care guidance. Please contact your doctor or another healthcare professional if you have any queries about health care. Like any other program for weight loss or maintenance, speak with your doctor or other healthcare practitioner before starting the Atkins Diet. Dialysis patients shouldn't follow the Atkins Diet's weight loss phases. Results may differ for each individual.

Atkins Eggs Scrambled with Cheddar, Swiss Chard and Canadian Bacon3.6gNet Carbs
Prep Time: 5 Minutes
Style:American
Cook Time: 8 Minutes
Phase: Phase 2
Difficulty: Moderate
32.6g
Protein
Fat
1.2g
Fiber

482.9cal
Calories
COMPOSITION
Three tsp extra virgin olive oil
Swiss Chard, six cups
Six large (whole) eggs
Shredded Cheddar Cheese, 3/4 cup
Six ounces Canadian-Style Cured Bacon
DIRECTIONS
Cook Swiss chard in 1 tsp oil until it becomes soft and reduces in volume.
Lightly beat eggs and pour into pan with Swiss chard. Mixing with a spatula, cook the eggs until they set.
Top with shredded Cheddar cheese and Canadian bacon, or mix it all in and fry it all at once.

Atkins Mushroom Scramble 4gNet Carbs
11.7g
Protein
14.2g
Fat
0.8g
Fiber
192.9cal
Calories

COMPOSITION
1 cup of stems and pieces of mushroom
half a cup of onions, chopped
three tsp Extra Virgin Olive Oil
14 ounces Stiff Silken Tofu
One cup of baby spinach
1/4 cup of cheddar cheese, shredded

Three teaspoons of grated Parmesan cheese
Four huge (whole) eggs
1/8 teaspoon dry thyme leaf powder
Eight cherry tomatoes
DIRECTIONS
1.Cook the white onion and mushrooms in the oil in a big, nonstick skillet over medium-high heat until they are tender, about 3 minutes.
2.Cook for a further three minutes after adding the tofu and spinach.
3.Cook until the egg is set, stirring in the tomatoes, eggs, Parmesan, and Cheddar cheeses along with 1/8 tsp thyme.
Serve right away.

RECIPE 3

Coffee cake with cinnamon crumbles
24 serving s
Ingredients:
First Step
two cups of flour
1/2 cup of brown sugar, tightly packed
1/2 cup of sugar, granulated
2 tablespoons McCormick® Ground Cloves
1 cup (2 sticks) cold butter, cut into chunks
One box, with two layers white cake mix
One egg
1 cup sour cream
1/4 cup (1/2 stick) butter, melted
1 teaspoon
INSTRUCTIONS
1
Preheat oven to 350°F. Mix flour, sugars and cinnamon in large bowl. Cut in cold butter with pastry blender or 2 knives until mixture resembles coarse crumbs. Set aside.
2
Beat cake mix, egg, sour cream, melted butter and vanilla in large bowl with electric mixer on medium speed about 1 minute or just until mixed.

3.spread evenly in greased and floured 13x9-inch baking pan. Sprinkle evenly with topping mixture.

4..Bake 30 to 35 minutes or until cake pulls away from sides of pan. Cool on wire rack. Cut into squares to serve.

TIPS AND TRICKS

Blueberry Crumb Cake: Prepare topping and batter as directed. Spread batter in baking pan. Sprinkle with 1 cup blueberries, then the topping mixture. Bake 45 minutes.

Atkins Almond Raspberry Smoothie10.3gNet Carbs

Prep Time: 5 Minutes

Style:American

Cook Time: 0 Minutes

Phase: Phase 2

Difficulty: Moderate

4 SERVING

INGREDIENTS

4 ounces Greek Yogurt - Plain (Container)

1/2 cup Red Raspberries

20 each wholes Blanched & Slivered Almonds

1/2 cup Pure Almond Milk - Unsweetened Original

DIRECTIONS

Feel free to experiment with other berries and nuts to make your own protein-rich smoothie. Make sure the frozen raspberries you use don't have any extra sugar.

In a blender, combine the yogurt, almond milk, raspberries, and almonds; process until smooth and creamy.

Atkins Keto Eggs with Avocado and Tomato4gNet Carbs

Prep Time: Minutes

Style:American

Cook Time: 5 Minutes

Phase: Phase 1

Difficulty: Moderate

2 SERVING *

14.8g
Protein
23.4g
Fat
6.6g
Fiber
302.5cal
Calories

INGREDIENTS
2 large Eggs (Whole)
1/2 medium whole (2-3/5" diameter) Red Tomatoes
1/2 fruit without skin and seed California Avocados
DIRECTIONS
Cook an egg whatever you'd like.
Cut the avocado and tomato into slices.
Eggs, avocado, and tomato are layered. If desired, add some chopped green
onions or paprika.

Atkins Keto Turkey Breakfast Meatloaf2.9gNet Carbs
Prep Time: 15 Minutes
Style:American
Cook Time: 55 Minutes
Phase: Phase 1

8 SERVINGS *
38.8g
Protein

17.1g
Fat

2.4g
Fiber

340.4cal
Calories

INGREDIENTS

1 10 oz package Frozen Chopped Spinach
4 stalk, medium (7-1/2" - 8" long) Celery
1 medium (approx 2-3/4" long, 2-1/2" diameter) Sweet Red Peppers
24 ounce raw (yield after cooking) Turkey Breakfast Sausage
1 1/2 pounds Ground Turkey
6 large Eggs (Whole)
1 small Onion
1/2 tsp, ground Thyme (Dried)
1 medium (approx 2-3/4" long, 2-1/2" diameter) Green Sweet Pepper
1/8 teaspoon Nutmeg (Ground)
1/8 tablespoon Red or Cayenne Pepper

DIRECTIONS

Preheat oven to 350°F.

Thaw the spinach and coarsely chop. Dice the celery, bell peppers and white onion.

Combine the ground turkey sausage and turkey, spinach, celery, bell peppers and onion until thoroughly mixed.

Add the eggs, thyme, cayenne, nutmeg, 1/2 teaspoon of garlic powder (if desired) and season with salt and freshly ground black pepper.

Distribute evenly and place in two standard quick bread pans (4x9 inches).

Bake until cooked through and browned on top; about 55-65 minutes.

Serve immediately or freeze in individual portions for up to 2 months.

Atkins Keto French Toast Casserole5.4gNet Carbs
Prep Time: 45 Minutes
Style:American
Cook Time: 80 Minutes
Phase: Phase
8 SERVINGS
13.8g
Protein5
36.7g

Fat
9.5g
Fiber

449.5cal
Calories

INGREDIENTS
14 large Eggs (Whole)
3 tablespoons Xylitol
10 tablespoons Unsalted Butter Stick
1 cup Organic High Fiber Coconut Flour
1 1/2 teaspoons Baking Powder (Straight Phosphate, Double Acting)
3/4 teaspoon Salt
1 cup Heavy Cream
1 cup Coconut Milk Unsweetened
1 teaspoon Cinnamon
1/4 teaspoon Nutmeg (Ground)
1/2 cup Sugar Free Maple Flavored Syrup
DIRECTIONS
1.While it's not required, it's ideal to prepare the bread part of this dish at least one day in advance (a week works excellent).

2.Turn the oven on to 350°F. Grease an 8 x 4-inch bread pan. Put aside.
In a medium bowl, whisk together 8 eggs, 1 tablespoon xylitol, and melted butter.
3.Blend the coconut flour, baking powder, and one-third teaspoon of salt using a sieve. Blend in the addition to the egg mixture until it thickens. Bake for 35 to 40 minutes, or until the sides become golden brown and pull away from the pan. After letting it cool in the pan for ten minutes, move it to a wire rack and let it cool for a total of thirty minutes. If baking ahead of time, chill the baked goods and store them in the refrigerator for up to two weeks in an airtight container or zip-top bag. If using right away, cool completely, then break into 1-inch pieces and transfer to a small casserole dish or the same pan you used to bake the bread.
4.Mix six eggs, heavy cream, coconut milk (you may use water or soy milk in place of the coconut milk), two tablespoons xylitol, nutmeg, cinnamon, and a dash of salt in a

medium-sized bowl. Cover the bread with the mixture and bake at 350°F for 50 minutes, or until the center is set. Divide into 8 portions and serve right away, covering each with 2 teaspoons of sugar-free pancake syrup (or roughly 1/3 cup for the entire casserole).

Atkins Eggs Scrambled with Zucchini, Cheddar and Sour Cream3.6g
Net Carbs
Prep Time: 10 Minutes
Style:American
Cook Time: 10 Minutes
Phase: Phase 1
Difficulty: Moderate
1 SERVING
21.1g
Protein
28.9g
Fat
0.67g
Fiber
361.9cal
Calories

INGREDIENTS
2 large Eggs (Whole)
2 tablespoons Sour Cream (Cultured)
1 teaspoon Extra Virgin Olive Oil
1/2 cup chopped Zucchini
1/4 cup shredded Cheddar Cheese
DIRECTIONS
Whisk together the sour cream and eggs lightly. Put aside.
In a skillet, preheat the heat to medium-high. Sauté the zucchini for two minutes on low heat in oil.
Cheese and the egg-sour cream mixture should be added to the pan and scrambled until cooked through.

Greek Easter Bread Recipe 6.5 net carb
Prep Time: 20 Minutes
Style:Mediterranean/Greek
Cook Time: 45 Minutes
Phase: Phase 2
14 servings
18.2g
Protein
11.6g
Fat
2.9g
Fiber
207.9cal
Calories
INGREDIENTS
4 2/3 large Eggs (Whole)
1 1/4 teaspoons Vinegar
1 1/4 packet (2.5 teaspoons) Active Dry Yeast
3 cups Whole Grain Soy Flour
4 2/3 ounces Vital Wheat Gluten
1 3/4 teaspoons Baking Powder (Sodium Aluminum Sulfate, Double Acting)
1/4 teaspoon Salt
4 2/3 tablespoons Butter
1 1/4 large Egg Yolks
1/4 cup Sucralose Based Sweetener (Sugar Substitute)
1 1/4 teaspoons Orange Zest
2/3 teaspoon Cinnamon
1/8 cup sliced Almonds
DIRECTIONS
1.For the eggs: Hard boil the eggs and then transfer them to a big enough stainless steel
dish to stay in a single layer. Add 1 tablespoon red food coloring, 1 cup water, and
vinegar and bring to a boil. Pour over eggs; leave for at least five minutes to let color to
seep into the egg shells. Take the eggs out of the dish and place them on a rack to dry.

2.Regarding bread: Use parchment paper to line a baking sheet. Sprinkle the yeast into 1/2 cup of warm water to activate it, then watch it froth. Put aside. In a large basin, combine soy flour, wheat gluten, baking powder, and salt. Combine one cup of warm water, yeast water, egg yolk, melted butter, sugar replacement, orange peel, and cinnamon. Blend with a spoon to create a soft dough after adding to the flour mixture. Knead manually for one minute. Shape the dough into a 6 × 8 rectangle and cut it into 3 lengthwise pieces. Roll each strip into a about 22–24-inch rope. Braide the strips, working straight onto the baking sheet. Form braid into circular with diameter of 10 to 12 inches.

3.Place eggs equally spaced along the braid. Place a plastic cover over it and let it rise for one to two hours, or until its mass has doubled. About fifteen minutes before the dough is done rising, preheat the oven to 350°F. Lightly coat dough with the leftover egg white (from the yolk) and scatter almonds on top.

4.Bake for 45 to 50 minutes, or until firm to the touch and golden brown. Take out of the oven and place on a wire rack to cool fully. Yields 12 servings.

LUNCH RECIPE

RECIPE 1

Atkins Low Carb Ranch fries string cheese 2,4g Carbs
Prep Time: 35 Minutes
Style:American
Cook Time: 4 Minutes
Phase: Phase 2
Difficulty: Moderate
5 SERVINGS *
10.9g
Protein
6.8g
Fat
0.9g
Fiber
167.7cal
Calories
INGREDIENTS
5 eas string mozzarella cheese
1 tablespoon almond flour, super finely ground, gluten free
1 lrg raw egg
1/2 tablespoon tap water
1 bag Atkins Ranch Protein Chips
4 teaspoons olive oil
1 teaspoon fresh young green scallions, chopped
DIRECTIONS
1.Halve the string cheese. Transfer the almond flour into one of
three small dishes. Whisk
the egg and water in the next bowl. Put the crumbled chips in
the final bowl. 2.One by
one, gently dust each string cheese slice with almond flour,
dunk it in the egg mixture,

and then cover it with crumbled chips. Put every covered string cheese onto a platter and
allow it to freeze for half an hour.
3,For at least three minutes, preheat the air fryer to 375°F.
4.Take the cheese sticks out of the freezer and spritz them well with olive oil. Arrange in
a single layer into the air fryer and cook for 3–4 minutes, or until the coating is golden
but not burnt and the cheese is melted.Take out of the air fryer and serve warm with a
scallion garnish. Two cheese sticks are included with each dish.

Atkins Vegan Keto Coconut Protein Shake1.3gNet Carbs
Prep Time: 5 Minutes
Style:American
Cook Time: 0 Minutes
Phase: Phase 1
Difficulty: Moderate
3 SERVING *
24.4g
Protein
5.6g
Fat
1g
Fiber
158.7cal
Calories
INGREDIENTS
1 cup Coconut Milk Unsweetened
1 ounce Protein Technologies International ProPlus Soy Protein Isolate
1/2 teaspoon Vanilla Extract
DIRECTIONS
For non-vegans or vegetarians, whey protein powder may be used instead; just add 1g
NC to the total NC content.
In a blender, combine all ingredients and 2-4 ice cubes (depending on desired thickness).
Think about substituting or adding coconut extract for the vanilla.
Mix well and taste.

Atkins Keto Crockpot Reuben Dip

2gNet Carbs

Prep Time: 10 Minutes
Style:American
Cook Time: 10 Minutes
Phase: Phase 1
Difficulty: Moderate
8 SERVINGS 5.5g
Protein
12.3g
Fat
0.4g
Fiber
141.7cal
Calories

COMPOSITION

Half a cup of Swiss cheese, shredded
Half a cup of canned sauerkraut, including liquid and solid
Cream cheese, 4 ounces
Half a cup of Cultured Sour Cream
Three tsp Original Stone Ground Mustard, ground
One-third spoonful of sauce with horseradish
two tsp Ketchup without sugar
4 ounces Brisket of corned beef (cured)

DIRECTIONS

Cut up Swiss cheese. Empty the sauerkraut.
Mix the softened cream cheese, sour cream, mustard, horseradish, and unsweetened
ketchup together in a small saucepan until well blended. Add the sauerkraut, cheddar, and
corned meat. Stir to evenly distribute all components.
Cook over medium heat until well warmed through and the cheese melts. Before serving,
put into a small 2-cup crockpot and let it remain warm for approximately ten minutes.
Alternatively, you may put it in an oven-safe bowl and cook it for half an hour at 350°F.
Serve right away. Accompany with other veggies or celery stalks.

Atkins Vegan "Ham," "Cream Cheese" and Dill Pickle Roll-Ups9.3gNet Carbs
Prep Time: 5 Minutes
Style:American
Cook Time: 0 Minutes
Phase: Phase 2
Difficulty: Moderate
7 SERVINGS
21.9g
Protein
11.7g
Fat
2.7g
Fiber
230.8cal
Calories
INGREDIENTS
9 1/8 servings Meatless Deli Ham
7 servings Vegan Gourmet Cream Cheese
14 spears Pickles
DIRECTIONS
Arrange two pieces of "ham." Cover them with an even layer of "cream cheese". Roll up
the pickle spear, placing it on one end. If needed, firmly secure with a toothpick.
Proceed with the remaining components.
Atkins Mini Mexican Pizza Squares 3g
Net Carbs
Prep Time: 15 Minutes
Style:American
Cook Time: 10 Minutes
Phase: Phase 2
10 SERVINGS
15.7g
Protein
9.8g
Fat

1.8g
Fiber
168.9cal
Calories
INGREDIENTS
10 servings Atkins Low Carb Wheat Bread
1 1/2 tablespoons Light Olive Oil
1 cup shredded Monterey Jack Cheese
4 ounces Salsa
2 large Scallions or Spring Onions
6 each Black Olives
1 ounce Cilantro
DIRECTIONS
1.Make Atkins Low Carb Wheat Bread with the Atkins recipe. Ten servings will be
required.
Preheat the oven to 400°F.
2.Remove the bread's crusts (save to make bread crumbs). Toast the bread
lightly after
brushing one side with olive oil. Divide every slice into four parts. On a baking
sheet,
arrange the squares.
3.Spoon a little tablespoon of salsa over each square of toast after the cheese
has been
divided. Add chopped olives and green onions on top.
4.Bake the cheese for 10 minutes, or until bubbly. Top the pizza squares with 2
tablespoons of finely chopped cilantro.
Serve right away.
COOKING ADVICE
Throwing a party? Consider which dishes you can prepare ahead of time and
which ones
require fresh ingredients on the same day when organizing your low-carb spread.

RECIPE 2

Atkins Strawberries and Walnuts5.1gNet Carbs
Prep Time: 5 Minutes
Style:American
Cook Time: 0 Minutes

Phase: Phase 2
Difficulty: Moderate
44.7g
Protein
18.7g
Fat
3g
Fiber
202.9cal
Calories
INGREDIENTS
1/3 cup sliced Strawberries
1 oz (14 halves) English Walnuts
DIRECTIONS
Add the strawberries and walnut halves together. or consume food separately. Have fun!
COOKING ADVICE
We adore the thought of personalizing this recipe to suit your tastes! Just be careful to
monitor the net carbs if you add any ingredients.

Atkins Keto Buffalo Chicken Wings1.8gNet Carbs
44.1g
Protein
70.8g
Fat
0.2g
Fiber
829.2cal
Calories
INGREDIENTS

1 large Egg (Whole)
1 tablespoon Tap Water
1/2 teaspoon Salt
1/2 teaspoon Celery salt
1/2 teaspoon Black Pepper
1/2 teaspoon Garlic Powder
32 ounces Chicken Wing with bone and skin

16 tablespoons Mayonnaise (Hellman's Real)
1/2 cup Sour Cream (Cultured)
1 medium (4-1/8" long) Scallions or Spring Onions
1/3 cup, crumbled Blue or Roquefort Cheese
/2 fluid ounce Fresh Lemon Juice
1 each Garlic, clove
1/2 cup Frank's Redhot Buffalo Wings Sauce
1/4 cup Butter, unsalted
DIRECTIONS
1.Turn the oven on to 450°F.
Using a fork, thoroughly combine the egg and water in a large bowl until frothy; set
aside. Mix the salt, pepper, garlic powder, and celery salt in a small bowl.
2.Make sure to coat each chicken wing uniformly after dipping it in the egg wash.
Transfer to a sizable baking sheet with a rim. Evenly distribute the seasonings on the
chicken's two sides. Bake the wings for thirty minutes, rotating them halfway through.
3.To make the dipping sauce, combine mayonnaise, sour cream, blue cheese, chopped
scallions, lemon juice, and minced garlic clove while the wings are cooking. Wait for the
wings to finish cooking.
4.Stir the butter and wing sauce together in a small pan over medium heat until the butter
melts. To keep warm until needed, turn down the heat.
5.To crisp the skin, turn the oven up to high broil and broil for two to three minutes on
each side. Take out of the oven, then brush each piece with the wing sauce, plate, and
serve hot with dipping sauce.
COOKING ADVICE
Try our Ranch Dressing recipe for an additional dipping sauce option.
Atkins Keto Eggless Tofu Salad4.1gNet Carbs
Prep Time: 10 Minutes
Style:American

Cook Time: 0 Minutes
Phase: Phase 1
Difficulty: Moderate
4 SERVINGS *
7.6g
Protein
21g
Fat
1.1g
Fiber
256.1cal
Calories
INGREDIENTS
14 ounces Firm Silken Tofu
2 stalk, medium (7-1/2" - 8" long) Celery
1/8 cup chopped Young Green Onions
1 medium Pickle
2 cloves Garlic
4 tablespoons Parsley
8 tablespoons Original Vegenaise
4 teaspoons Dijon Mustard
1/8 teaspoon Turmeric (Ground)
1 teaspoon Salt
DIRECTIONS 1. Chop the pickle, onions, celery, and tofu.
Combine everything in a medium-sized bowl with the minced parsley and garlic.
Combine the Vegenaise, Dijon mustard, turmeric, and salt in a small blender and add it to
the tofu mixture. Toss until all of the dressing has been applied.
Add to Romaine lettuce leaves and roll up, or top a low-carb tortilla and enjoy as you
would egg salad.
COOKING ADVICE
Feel free to use any type of lettuce you prefer for this recipe; the net carbohydrate content
should be fairly low.

Atkins Chili Spiced "Tortilla" Wraps1.4gNet Carbs
Prep Time: 5 Minutes
Style:American
Cook Time: 15 Minutes
Phase: Phase 2
9 SERVINGS4.5g
Protein
4.3g
Fat
2.5g
Fiber
73.7cal
Calories
INGREDIENTS
6 3/4 tablespoons Organic High Fiber Coconut Flour
1 2/3 teaspoons Chili Powder
2 1/4 tablespoons Organic 100% Whole Ground Golden Flaxseed Meal
1/4 teaspoon Salt
1 1/8 cups Coconut Milk Unsweetened
4 1/2 whites Egg White
2 1/4 each Egg
1 1/8 teaspoons Xylitol
2 1/4 teaspoons Olive Oil
DIRECTIONS
1. In a small bowl, mix together coconut flour, chili powder, flax meal, and salt. Put
aside.
Beat together the whole egg, egg whites, coconut milk, and sugar substitute. After
adding and combining the flour mixture, let it sit for five minutes.
2. Set a 350°F electric griddle. Apply a thin layer of oil to the skillet. Transfer a quarter of
a cup of batter onto the griddle and use it to form a 5-inch tortilla that is no thicker than
1/4 of an inch. Cook on the first side for at least 7 minutes, or until a spatula can be used
to flip it without it falling apart. 3. After 3 minutes, flip the food over and continue
cooking until it's cooked through and the edges start to brown. Continue, drizzling oil in
between each batch, until four tortilla wraps are formed.

4. Arrange the cooked tortillas with a paper towel in between each one. Eat warm
store in the refrigerator in an airtight container with paper towels between layers for up to
1 week. Before serving, reheat in a dry skillet over medium-high heat for 30 seconds on
each side. Or freeze for up to three months. A single tortilla represents a single serving.
Not even an electric griddle? You can prepare these on top of the stove. One teaspoon of
oil and a large nonstick skillet are heated over medium-high heat. Lower the temperature
to medium and transfer the batter into the pan with a 1/4 cup measure, spreading it out to
form a 5-inch tortilla. Bake for 3 to 5 minutes, or until the top is completely set and the
bottom is golden brown. Turn and cook for a further one to three minutes. Continue with
the final three tortillas.

Atkins Cardamom Butter Cookies2gNet Carbs
Prep Time: 45 Minutes
Style:American
Cook Time: 10 Min
Difficulty: Moderate
25 SERVINGS3.8g
Protein
7g
Fat
0.9g
Fiber
86cal
Calories
INGREDIENTS
1 1/2 servings
1/2 cup Blanched Almond Flour
1/4 teaspoon Baking Powder (Straight Phosphate, Double Acting)
1/2 teaspoon Salt
10 tablespoons Unsalted Butter Stick
1/2 cup Sucralose Based Sweetener (Sugar Substitute)
1 large Egg (Whole)
1 tablespoon Tap Water
2 teaspoons Vanilla Extract
1 teaspoon confectioners erythritol sweetener

3/4 tsp, ground Cardamom
8 teaspoons tap water
1/8 teaspoon cardamom, ground
DIRECTIONS
1. For this recipe, please use the Atkins recipe for the sweet version of the Soy-Free Flour
Mix with Vanilla Whey Protein. You will need 1 1/2 cups of the mix (1 1/2 servings,
half a recipe) for this recipe. You will need to make the necessary adjustments if you
decide to upsize or downsize the recipe's serving size.
2. In a medium bowl, mix almond flour, baking powder, Atkins Soy-Free Flour Mix, and
salt.
Cream room temperature butter and sugar substitute in big bowl of stand mixer until
fluffy and light. Mix the egg, water, vanilla, and ¾ teaspoon of cardamom together at
room temperature. Beat on medium speed until well combined, scraping down the
sides
of the bowl as needed. The mixture may appear watery. Gradually add flour mixture
and
mix on low speed until dough comes together.
3. Place the dough in a resealable bag, wrap it in parchment paper, and refrigerate for
half
an hour.
Preheat the oven to 350°F. Use parchment paper to line two baking sheets.
Roll out dough between sheets of parchment paper to a thickness of ¼ inch; cut
shapes
with small cookie cutters or a sharp knife. Try again after 10 minutes in the freezer if
the
rolled-out dough is too sticky or isn't holding the shapes well. About fifty nine-gram
raw
dough cookies should be produced. Bake for ten minutes, or until the bottoms are
golden;
during the last few minutes, keep a close eye on them to make sure they don't burn.
After
five minutes of cooling on baking sheets, move the cookies to a wire rack to finish
cooling.
5. While the cookies cool, make a paste in a small bowl by combining 1/8 teaspoon
cardamom, 8 teaspoons water, and confectioners erythritol with a fork. Evenly drizzle
icing over cooled cookies, letting them dry before storing.
For up to a week, keep stored in an airtight container. A serving consists of two
cookies,
or 14 g of cooked dough.

Atkins Raspberry Soy Frappe 10.6gNet Carbs

8.5g

Protein

4.8g

Fat

10.1g

Fiber

148cal

Calories

COMPOSITION

Half a cup of frozen raspberries without sugar

1 cup of unsweetened organic soy milk and 2 packets Packets of No Calorie Sweetener

1/4 tspn Whole Almond Extract

DIRECTIONS

Blend all ingredients until smooth on high speed.

After adding three ice cubes or half a cup of crushed ice, blend once more until smooth.

Have fun!

COOKING ADVICE

You can adjust the serving settings above to indicate the necessary quantity of

ingredients, regardless of whether you're cooking for one person or a large family.

DINNER RECIPES

Atkins Keto Steaks with Green Onion and Caper Sauce 0.8gNet Carbs
Prep Time: 10 Minutes
Style:Other
Cook Time: 8 Minutes
Phase: Phase 2
Difficulty: Moderate
4 SERVINGS *
49.6g
Protein
28.9g
Fat
0.7g
Fiber
474.7cal
Calories
COMPOSITION
Two large spring onions or scallions
4 tablespoons of capers, drained
Three tsp Dijon Mustard
One-third cup red wine vinegar
One-fourth cup of extra virgin olive oil
two tsp of parsley
A 24-oz rib-eye steak
DIRECTIONS
1. Set the broiler pan to 4 inches from the heat source and preheat the broiler.
2. Add salt and pepper to the steaks, then cook them for the desired doneness
(medium-rare is, roughly, 3 to 4 minutes per side).

3. Make sauce while the steaks are cooking: Mix the mustard, onions, capers, and red
wine vinegar together in a small bowl. Drizzle in olive oil gradually and whisk until a
slight thickening occurs. Add the parsley and season with salt and pepper to taste.
4. Before serving, drizzle sauce over the steaks.

Atkins Keto Chili-Beef Kebabs1.3gNet Carbs
Prep Time: 30 Minutes
Style:Other
Cook Time: 12 Minutes
Phase: Phase 1
Difficulty: Moderate
8 SERVINGS *
23.1g
Protein
19.9g
Fat
0.8g
Fiber
283.4cal
Calories
COMPOSITION
Three teaspoons of garlic, two tablespoons of canola vegetable oil
One tablespoon of chili powder
a single tsp salt
1/8 tsp red or black pepper Chili
Two lbs. of beef Top Sirloin, Choice Grade, Trimmed to 1/8" Fat
Eight medium-sized (4-1/8-inch-long) spring onions
two tsp of parsley

DIRECTIONS
In a bowl, mix together oil, minced garlic, chili powder, salt, and red pepper. To coat, add
the beef tossing. Let it marinate for one hour.
If using, soak bamboo skewers in water fifteen minutes before grilling, and heat your grill
to medium.
Alternatively, skewer pieces of beef and halved green onions. Kebabs should be cooked
through after 10 to 15 minutes of grilling, turning them occasionally. After adding
parsley, serve.

Atkins Italian Chopped Salad8.2gNet Carbs
Prep Time: 20 Minutes
Style:Italian
Cook Time: 0 Minutes
Phase: Phase 1
2 SERVINGS *
29.6g
Protein
28.4g
Fat
4.6g
Fiber
420.4cal
INGREDIENTS
2 tablespoons Red Wine Vinegar
1 tablespoon Basil, fresh, chopped
1 tablespoon Parmesan Cheese, grated
1 teaspoon Dijon Mustard
1 tablespoon Olive Oil
1/2 cup Snap Peas, in pod, fresh, chopped
1 cup Cucumber, raw, sliced
10 each Cherry or Grape Tomato
2 ounces Mozzarella Cheese, fresh balls
1/2 package (4 oz) Hard Salami

4 ounces Chicken Roasted, dark and light meat
4 cups Romaine, raw, shredded
1 cup Baby Spinach
DIRECTIONS
Whisk the mustard with the vinegar, Parmesan, and chopped basil. Whisk the oil into the
vinaigrette gradually. Put aside.
Chop the cooked chicken, salami, cucumber, tomatoes, mozzarella cheese, and peas into
bite-sized pieces to prepare the vegetables.
Combine the spinach and romaine lettuce with the dressing. Add the cheese, meats, and
chopped vegetables on top. Serve right away.
COOKING ADVICE
Feel free to use any type of lettuce you prefer for this recipe; the net carbohydrate content
should be fairly low

.

Atkins Turkey Tacos7.5gNet Carbs
Prep Time: 10 Minutes
Style:American
Cook Time: 10 Minutes
Phase: Phase 2
6 SERVINGS
39.5g
Protein
17.7g
Fat
4.8g
Fiber
356.7cal
Calories
INGREDIENTS
3 tablespoons Light Olive Oil
24 oz, boneless, cooked, skinlesses Turkey Cutlet
1 1/2 tablespoons Original Taco Seasoning Mix
1/2 cup Sour Cream (Cultured)

1/2 cup chopped Red Onions
1 1/2 ounces Cilantro (Coriander)
6 tortillas Low Carb Tortillas
3/4 medium (approx 2-3/4" long, 2-1/2" diameter) Green Sweet Pepper
3 ounces Salsa   .DIRECTIONS
1. In a large skillet, heat 1 tablespoon (3 teaspoons) oil over medium-high heat. Taco
seasoning should be added to the turkey cutlets before they are cooked through, which
should take two minutes on each side. After moving the turkey to a chopping board, cut it
into strips.
2. Fill skillet with sour cream, onion, and cilantro. Simmer for 3 minutes or until mixture
is well heated and onions are starting to soften.
3. Put the turkey strips back in the skillet with any juices that have collected, toss to coat,
and turn off the heat.
4. In a medium skillet over high heat, heat 1 teaspoon oil until it's very hot, then proceed
to make each taco. Add tortilla and cook until light golden brown, one minute on each
side. Eliminate and pour away surplus oil onto paper towels. Top with 1/4 of the pepper
strips and 1 tablespoon of salsa after placing 1/4 of the filling on one half of the tortilla
and folding it over. Use the remaining tortillas to repeat the entire process.

Atkins Curried Fish and Red Peppers Over Broccoli8.1gNet Carbs
43.3g
Protein
17.5g
Fat
0.9g
Fiber
354.3cal
Calories
INGREDIENTS
32 ounces Tilapia
6 cup flowerets Broccoli Flower Clusters

1 1/2 cups Coconut Cream, canned
1/2 tablespoon Roasted Red Chili Paste
2 teaspoons Ginger
1 1/2 tablespoons Fish Sauce
3 teaspoons Sucralose Based Sweetener (Sugar Substitute)
3 cups sliced Red Sweet Pepper
1/2 fluid ounce Fresh Lime Juice
DIRECTIONS
Season fish with a small amount of salt and freshly ground black pepper. Put aside.
Get a medium pot filled with water that has a steamer basket ready to boil. After the
water reaches a boil, steam the broccoli for five to ten minutes, or until it is crisp-
tender.
As the broccoli steams, get the fish and sauce ready.
Add the coconut milk, chili paste, minced ginger, lime juice, fish sauce, granulated
sugar
substitute, and bell peppers to a large sauté pan set over medium-high heat. After
mixing
the sauce ingredients and bringing it to a boil, add the fish. Fish should be cooked by
basting it every two to three minutes with the sauce until the flesh is opaque and flake
easily. After removing the fish to a plate, reduce the sauce over medium heat until it
slightly thickens. Rewarm the fish in the pan for two to three minutes, squeeze in the
lime
juice, and serve right away over the broccoli.

Atkins Double Mushroom Soup5.4gNet Carbs
Prep Time: 35 Minutes
Style:American
Cook Time: 45 Minutes
Phase: Phase 2
6 SERVINGS *
12.3g
Protein
16g
Fat
1.2g
Fiber
217.7cal

INGREDIENTS

Five dried porcini mushroom pieces

Four cans (10.75 ounces), cooked according to the recipe Consomme, Bouillon, or Chicken Broth

Stick of three tablespoons unsalted butter

One tiny onion

Dozen ounces Parts of mushrooms and stems

three tsp Garlic

three tsp Mixture of Atkins flour

One tsp of thyme

One-fourth teaspoon ground nutmeg

Half a cup of heavy cream

DIRECTIONS

1. To make the Atkins flour mix needed for this recipe, follow the Atkins recipe. Pour 14 1/2 ounces of chicken broth over the porcinis in a bowl and let stand for 30 minutes. Pour off the soaking liquid and reserve. Chop porcinis coarsely and reserve.

2. In a sauce pot over medium heat, melt the butter. Saute the button mushrooms and diced onion for ten minutes. Simmer the minced garlic for an additional thirty seconds.

Stir in three tablespoons of Atkins Flour Mix; cook for two minutes.

3. Gradually mix in the nutmeg, thyme, reserved porcini liquid, and the remaining 29 ounces of chicken broth. After turning the heat up to high and bringing it to a boil, lower it to medium-low and simmer for five minutes. Add chopped porcinis to soup and simmer until softened, about 10 more minutes.

4. Transfer half of the soup to a pot after blending it smooth in a food processor or blender. Simmer soup for three minutes after adding cream. To taste, add salt and pepper for seasoning.

COOKING ADVICE

You may easily portion out soup and freeze it for a busy night later, didn't you know that?

When ready to reheat, warm in a pot on the stovetop with a splash of water or in a microwave.

Atkins Roasted Vegetable Soup 6.7gNet Carbs
Prep Time: 20 Minutes
Style:Other
Cook Time: 75 Minutes
Phase: Phase 2
8 SERVINGS *
4.9g
Protein
17.3g
Fat
5.6g
Fiber
212.3cal
Calories
INGREDIENTS
Four ripe tomatoes crimson tomatoes
Two unpeeled eggplant (roughly 1.4 lbs.) eggplant
Four cloves Garlic
three tsp Mild Olive Oil
1/4 teaspoon dried marjoram
Two cans of 14.5 ounces Consomme, Bouillon, or Chicken Broth
One cup of heavy cream
three-quarter teaspoon Salt
Half a teaspoon of black pepper
Six large spring onions, or shallots
DIRECTIONS
1.Preheat the oven to 400°F.
In a shallow roasting pan, arrange the tomatoes, eggplants, green onions, and garlic. Toss
with marjoram and oil. Roast for 40 minutes, turning occasionally, or until vegetables are
soft and beginning to turn brown. After the eggplants have cooled down sufficiently,
remove the pulp and place it in a large saucepot. Include the other vegetables.
2. Mix into broth. Bring over high heat to a boil. Vegetables should be simmered for 35
minutes on low heat to become extremely tender. Nice.

3. Blend soup in batches using a blender. Put the soup back in the saucepot. Add cream,
pepper, and salt, and stir. Warm up thoroughly.

Atkins Keto Smoky Tuna Tomato 2.3gNet Carbs
Prep Time: 10 Minutes
Style:American
Cook Time: 0 Minutes
Phase: Phase 1
Difficulty: Moderate
2 SERVINGS *
26.8g
Protein
33.1g
Fat
1.1g
Fiber
421.3cal
Calories
COMPOSITION
One whole medium (2–3/5" in diameter) crimson tomato
Six ounces Can of Tuna in Water
One tablespoon of finely chopped chives
Six Tablespoons Genuine Mayonnaise
three tsp Actual Bacon Snacks
One half-ounce glass of fresh lemon juice
Each whole Chipotle en Adobo, half
1/8 teaspoon Salt
DIRECTIONS
1. Halve the tomato and remove the pulp and seeds. Sprinkle salt and pepper on top
(optional) and drizzle with a little olive oil.
Dice the chipotle pepper finely and transfer to a small bowl with the other ingredients
(drain the tuna first, of course). 2. After blending to incorporate, spoon tuna mixture into
tomato halves and serve.

COOKING ADVICE
Before serving, sprinkle with smoked paprika to give this naturally low-carb and keto
recipe a little more color and smokey flavor!

Atkins Keto Baked Tofu with Latin Marinade 5.6gNet Carbs
Prep Time: 5 Minutes
Style:Other
Cook Time: 30 Minutes
Phase: Phase 1
Difficulty: Moderate
1 SERVING *
12g
Protein
25.6g
Fat
0.4g
Fiber
299.1cal
Calories
INGREDIENTS
1 serving Keto Latin Marinade
6 ounces Firm Silken Tofu
DIRECTIONS
1. To make Latin Marinade, follow the Atkins recipe; you'll need 2 tablespoons.
2. Drain the tofu and use a paper towel to pat dry. After cutting into 1/4-inch strips,
marinate them.
3. Turn the oven on to 375° 3. If desired, marinate the tofu for at least thirty minutes.
On a flat pan that has been greased, bake for 15 minutes, then flip and continue baking
for another 15 minutes, or until golden brown and slightly crispy. To use on a salad or to
reheat for a warm meal, serve right away or store in the refrigerator for up to three days.

CHAPTER 7: DESSERTS

Atkins Keto Chocolate Pecan Shortbread Drops0.7gNet Carbs
Prep Time: 20 Minutes
Style:American
Cook Time: 14 Minutes
Phase: Phase
50 SERVINGS *
1.2g
Protein
4.9g
Fat
0.5g
Fiber
50.7cal
Calories
INGREDIENTS
16 tablespoons Unsalted Butter Stick
1/2 cup Sucralose Based Sweetener (Sugar Substitute)
1/2 teaspoon stevia sweetener
1 large Egg (Whole)
2 tablespoons Cream, heavy, liquid
1 teaspoon Vanilla Extract
3/4 cup(s) Soy flour, defatted (1 cup= 105g)
3 teaspoons Baking Powder (Straight Phosphate, Double Acting)
3 tablespoons Cocoa Powder
1/2 cup chopped Pecan Nuts

DIRECTIONS
1. Turn the oven on to 325°F.
Using an electric mixer, beat butter, stevia, and sucralose on medium speed for
approximately four minutes, or until light and fluffy. Reduce the speed to low
and mix in
the egg, cream, vanilla, and optional 1 tsp chocolate extract. After scraping
down the
sides of the bowl, stir in the soy flour, baking powder, cocoa powder, and
pecans until
just combined.
2. Spoon dough onto ungreased baking sheets in heaping teaspoonfuls. Cook
for 12 to 14
minutes, or until the cookies are firm. Allow to cool for one minute on the
sheets, then
move to wire racks to finish cooling.
COOKING ADVICE
We adore the thought of personalizing this recipe to suit your tastes! Just be
careful to
monitor the net carbs if you add any ingredients.

Atkins Walnut Blondies 5.2gNet Carbs
Prep Time: 20 Minutes
Style:American
Cook Time: 14 Minutes
Phase: Phase 3
12 SERVINGS *
8.7g
Protein
26.2g
Fat
2.1g
Fiber
286.5cal
Calories
INGREDIENTS
Chopped English walnuts, one cup
One cup Stick of unsalted butter
One cup of sugar substitute sweetener based on sucrose
One tsp vanilla extract
1 cup Soy Flour, Whole Grain
Half a cup of whole wheat pastry flour that has been stone-ground
Three huge (whole) eggs
One ounce of gluten made from vital wheat
One and a half tsp straight phosphate, double-acting baking powder

Half a teaspoon of cinnamon
Two portions of baking chocolate squares without sweetener
DIRECTIONSSo
Preheat the oven to 325°F. On a sheet pan, toast the walnuts for 8 to 10 minutes. Once
cooled, finely chop them. Put aside.
2. Wrap two inches of aluminum foil around the short sides of a 13 by 9-inch baking pan.
Oil the foil and keep it aside.
3. In a large basin, whisk together butter, sugar substitute, eggs, and vanilla extract. Mix
the flours, baking powder, gluten, and cinnamon in a separate dish, then thoroughly mix
them into the butter mixture. Add walnuts and stir. Evenly spread into the pan that has
been prepared. Bake for 12 to 14 minutes, or until puffed and set and a toothpick inserted
in center comes out clean (top will not brown).
4. Allow the pan to cool fully on a wire rack. Over the whole surface of the brownies,
drizzle chocolate in thin lines. Let stand for about an hour or until set. (You can make the
recipe up to this stage, wrap it in plastic wrap, and leave it overnight at room temperature.)
5. Remove the brownies from the pan by firmly grasping both ends of the foil and set
them on a work surface. After cutting into 12 pieces, serve.

Atkins Vanilla Mousse with Rhubarb Sauce7.5gNet Carbs
Prep Time: 15 Minutes
Style:American
Cook Time: 10 Minutes
Phase: Phase 2
Difficulty: Moderate
2 SERVINGS
7.3g
Protein
22.1g
Fat
1.9g
Fiber

253.7cal
Calories
INGREDIENTS
2 stalks Rhubarb
1/4 cup Tap Water
1 tablespoon Sugar Free Strawberry Jam
1/2 cup Heavy Cream
4 ounces Greek Yogurt - Plain (Container)
3 teaspoons Sucralose Based Sweetener (Sugar Substitute)
DIRECTIONS
1. To make the rhubarb sauce, put the rhubarb, water, and strawberry jam in a small
saucepan and heat it to a simmer over medium heat. Lower the heat to medium-low,
cover, and simmer for approximately 10 minutes, stirring now and again, until the
rhubarb takes on the consistency of sauce. Put aside to cool.
2. To make the vanilla mousse, whip the cream, 4 ounces of yogurt, and sugar substitute
in a mixing bowl on medium-high speed with an electric mixer until semi-firm
peaks form.. Set aside 1/4 cup mousse for the garnish.
3. To assemble: Place two wineglasses or martini glasses on the table. Evenly distribute
1/4 cup of mousse in the bottom of each glass using a spoon. Add 1 1/2 tablespoons of
rhubarb sauce on top of each. Spoon the leftover mousse into each glass, then garnish
with the remaining rhubarb. Evenly divide the 1/4 cup mousse that was set aside on top.

Atkins Strawberries with French Cream 6.4gNet Carbs
Prep Time: 10 Minutes
Style:French
Cook Time: 0 Minutes
Phase: Phase 2
Difficulty: Moderate
4 SERVINGS *
1.5g
Protein
13.1g
fat

150.4cal
Calories
INGREDIENTS
1/2 cup Heavy Cream
1 tablespoon Sucralose Based Sweetener (Sugar Substitute)
3 tablespoons Sour Cream (Cultured)
12 ounces fresh strawberries
DIRECTIONS 1. Beat cream and sugar substitute on high speed for 4 minutes, or until
soft peaks form.
2. Until completely combined, beat in sour cream. Accompany with berries.

Atkins Low Carb Irish Coffee1gNet Carbs
0.6g
Protein
7.3g
Fat
0g
Fiber
176cal
Calories
INGREDIENTS
36 ounces of fluid decaffeinated coffee
Spirits nine fluid ounces without ice
Three tsp of sugar substitute sweetener based on sucrose
A half-cup of thickened cream
DIRECTIONS
Pour out and reserve 4 ½ cups (36 fl oz) of coffee.
In a small saucepan, reheat the whiskey (9 fl oz, or 1 cup plus 2 teaspoons) over
medium-low heat; do not boil. Mix hot whiskey and powdered sugar into just-brewed
coffee.
Lightly beat heavy cream in the small bowl of an electric mixer set on medium speed
until soft peaks form.

Divide the coffee mixture into 6 cups, or slightly less than 1 cup per serving, or about 7 ½
fluid ounces per serving. Top each cup with a dollop of whipped cream (about 2
teaspoons per serving).

Atkins Atkins Pie Crust 3.6gNet Carbs
Prep Time: 65 Minutes
Style:American
Cook Time: 16 Minutes
Phase: Phase 3
8 SERVINGS *
8.6g
Protein
13.2g
Fat
1.3g
Fiber
168.2cal
Calories
INGREDIENTS
1/3 cup 100% Stone Ground Whole Wheat Pastry Flour
1/3 cup Whole Grain Soy Flour
2 ounces Vital Wheat Gluten
3 tablespoons Plain Wheat Germ
1/2 teaspoon Salt
1/2 cup Unsalted Butter Stick
1 tablespoon Tap Water
DIRECTIONS
1. Pulse the flours, butter, wheat germ, gluten, and salt in a food processor until the
mixture resembles coarse meal. Water should be added gradually while pulsing the dough
until it starts to come together. Transfer to a plastic wrap sheet, roll into a ball, and wrap
in plastic. Press into a 7-inch round and freeze for fifteen minutes.

2. Roll out the dough to a 12-inch circle between two sheets of plastic wrap; if necessary,
dust each side with 1/2 teaspoon of wheat gluten flour to make rolling easier. Take off the
top plastic sheet and turn the mixture over onto a 9-inch pie pan. Press the dough into the
center of the plate's sides and bottom. Take out the plastic, roll the edges under, and add
ornamental crimps. For fifteen minutes, let it cool in the freezer.
3. Follow the directions for the unbaked crust in your preferred recipe. Alternately,
preheat the oven to 400° F for a prebaked crust. Using a fork, prick the pie shell's edges
and bottom. Pie weights or dried beans can be used to partially fill a lined pie shell. Then,
flip the foil over to cover the pastry border. Bake for sixteen minutes. After removing the
weights and foil, bake for a further 4 to 6 minutes, or until golden. Loosely cover with
foil. Before using, let cool on a rack for 20 minutes.
4. Yields 8 portions.

Atkins Keto Coconut Thumbprints0.9gNet Carbs
Prep Time: 20 Minutes
Style:American
Cook Time: 8 Minutes
Phase: Phase 2
36 SERVINGS *
1.3g
Protein
5.7g
Fat
0.7g
Fiber
60cal
Calories
INGREDIENTS
2/3 cup, shelled (32 kernels) Brazil Nuts
1/2 cup Coconut, shredded, unsweetened
1/2 cup Whole Grain Soy Flour
2 1/2 tablespoons Sucralose Based Sweetener (Sugar Substitute)

1/2 cup Unsalted Butter Stick
1 large Egg (Whole)
1 large Egg Yolk
1 teaspoon Coconut Extract
3 tablespoons Sugar Free Seedless Blackberry Jam
DIRECTIONS
1. Turn the oven on to 375°F.
Pulse 1/2 cup coconut and nuts in a food processor for approximately one minute, or until
finely ground. Pulse to blend in the sugar replacement and soy flour.
2. Add the butter and pulse for a further 30 seconds or until the mixture resembles coarse
grain. Add the egg, yolk, and extract, and pulse for one minute, or until the dough just
comes together.
3. Scrape dough into bowl, cover, and refrigerate until somewhat set, at least three hours.
Create 36 spheres out of the dough, then place them on an ungreased baking sheet. Make
a depression in the middle of each ball, resembling a doughnut, by dipping your thumb
into warm water (don't press all the way through).
5. Spoon a ¼ teaspoon of jam into each depression. Bake for about 6 minutes, or until
brown. Allow to cool for one minute on the baking sheet, then move to wire racks to
finish cooling.

RECIPE 2

Atkins Coconut Pie
9.3gNet Carbs
Prep Time: 30 Minutes
Style:American
Cook Time: 20 Minutes
Phase: Phase 2
8 SERVINGS *
12.2g
Protein
41.3g
Fat
3.8g
Fiber

473.4cal
Calories
COMPOSITION
1 1/2 cups of extremely fine almond meal with skin
1 3/4 cups shredded, unsweetened coconut
3/4 cup Sugar Substitute Sweetener Based on Sucralose
One big egg white
1 tablespoon coconut oil
one and a quarter cups of coconut cream in a can
Half a cup of heavy cream
Six large (whole) eggs
One huge egg yolk
One tsp vanilla extract
One tsp of extract from coconut
1/4 tsp salt
DIRECTIONS
For crust
Preheat the oven to 350°F. Grease a 9-inch pie plate very lightly.
2.Combine almond meal, melted coconut oil, egg white, 1/4 cup sugar substitute, and one
cup shredded coconut. Add one to two tablespoons of water, a few drops at a time, if the
mixture is too dry to keep together, until it retains its shape when pressed together.
Form a crust by pressing equally onto the bottom and up the sides of the prepared pie
plate. For fifteen minutes, bake until gently browned. Take out of oven and place aside.
Increase oven temperature to 450°F.
For completing
3.Scald coconut milk and cream in a medium saucepan (in a heavy bottom pan over medium heat, warm the coconut milk combination stirring regularly until small bubbles
begin to form along the sides of the pan, or the milk reaches 180-185°); set aside to cool
slightly.
In a large bowl, with an electric mixer on medium speed (or with a wire whisk), beat eggs
and egg yolk until frothy. Beat in 1/2 cup sugar substitute, vanilla and coconut extract,
and salt. Slowly beat in warm coconut milk mixture.
4.Fold in all but 2 tablespoons of remaining coconut shreds (3/4 cup) and stir gently. Pour
filling into prepared crust, and sprinkle with the last 2 tablespoons coconut shreds. Bake 5
minutes at 450°F. Reduce temperature to 350°F and bake 15 minutes more. Watch the

crust in the last 10 minutes, adding a strip of foil around the edge if needed to prevent
burning. When the middle of the pie is easily cut with a knife and the internal
temperature hits 160°, the pie is done. Cool on a wire rack to room temperature, then
transfer to refrigerator to chill completely. Makes 8 servings.

Atkins Pear Tart 13.3gNet Carbs
Prep Time: 40 Minutes
Style:French
Cook Time: 30 Minutes
Phase: Phase 3
6 SERVINGS *
11.3g
Protein
32.5g
Fat
4.2g
Fiber
403.7cal
Calories
COMPOSITION
3/4 cup Soy Flour, Whole Grain
Nine tablespoons of sugar substitute made with sucrose
Four teaspoons of stick unsalted butter
One pound of cream cheese
One tablespoon of cultured sour cream
2 little pears (around 3 per pound) One fluid ounce of pear (no ice) bourbon
One-half tsp pure almond extract
Half a teaspoon ground ginger
Sugar-free apricot preserves, two tablespoons
One huge egg, whole
Two tsp tap water and one ounce of almonds

Directions
Set oven temperature to 350°F.
2. Regarding crust: Pulse the flour and two tablespoons of sugar substitute in a food
processor for approximately ten seconds. Add butter and process for 30 seconds or
until
mixture resembles coarse grain.
3. Add the sour cream and 3 ounces of cream cheese, and pulse for an additional 30
seconds or until the dough begins to come together. Press the dough into an
ungreased
10-tart pan, covering the bottom and the sides. While making the filling, prick the
dough with a fork approximately fifteen times and
place it in the freezer.
To be filled: Slices of pear should be uniformly divided after being combined with 1/4
teaspoon of almond essence, 1 tablespoon of sugar replacement, brandy or Cognac,
and
ginger in a small bowl.4. Set aside 4. In a large bowl, whisk 1/3 cup sugar substitute
and
8 ounces room temperature cream cheese on high speed for about 3 minutes, or until
smooth and creamy. Beat the egg and the remaining 1/4 teaspoon almond extract for
5
more minutes, scraping down the sides of the bowl as needed, until the mixture is
smooth.
Fill the chilled tart shell with the cream cheese mixture. Place pears in concentric
circles
that slightly overlap on top of the cream cheese mixture. Pour any remaining liquid
from
the pears evenly over the tart.
6. Bake until the cheese mixture is barely set, about 30 minutes. Take out of the oven
and
let cool on a wire rack.
Melt jam in a pan over medium heat with water. 7. By my Drizzle hot tart with almond
powder. Allow tart to cool fully before cutting.

Atkins Bittersweet Chocolate Brownie Drops 2.9gNet Carbs
Prep Time: 15 Minutes
Style:American
Cook Time: 10 Minutes
Phase: Phase 3
12 SERVINGS *
2.6g
Protein
9.3g
Fat

1.1g
Fiber
100cal
Calories
COMPOSITION
Two tsp of whole wheat pastry flour that has been stone ground
Two tablespoons of soy flour (whole grain)
1/4 teaspoon of double-acting, straight phosphate baking powder
Squares of baking chocolate without sugar, 3 ounces
Six Tablespoons Heavy Cream
2 tablespoons Unsalted Butter Stick
Two huge (whole) eggs
3/4 cup Sugar Substitute Sweetener Based on Sucralose
DIRECTIONS
1. Turn the oven on to 375°F. Use aluminum foil or parchment paper to line a
baking pan.
2. Combine 2 tablespoons flour, soy flour, and baking powder in a big bowl.
Melt the chocolate, cream, and butter in a microwave-safe bowl for one to two
minutes,
or until the butter is melted and the chocolate has softened. After two minutes,
let stand
and stir until smooth. This stage can also be completed on a cooktop.
3. Beat eggs and sugar substitute for three minutes on medium speed with an
electric
mixer, or until light and fluffy. Gradually beat the slightly warm chocolate
mixture into
the egg mixture until well-blended, about 1 minute. Reduce the speed of your
mixer to
low and quickly mix in the flour mixture.
4. Drop dough onto prepared sheet in gently rounded teaspoonfuls. Bake for 5–6
minutes,
or until the top is slightly soft but the center is set. Transfer to a wire rack to cool
completely.

Atkins Frozen Chocolate Fudge Tart5.9gNet Carbs
Prep Time: 210 Minutes
Style:American
Cook Time: 20 Minutes
Phase: Phase 2
12 SERVINGS *

29.4g
Fat
4.4g
Fiber
310.6cal
Calories
INGREDIENTS
half a serving
Five teaspoons of unsweetened cocoa powder You
Half a teaspoon of cinnamon
Seven tsp Sucralose-Based Sweetener (Sugar Alternative)
Four teaspoons of stick unsalted butter
Three ounces of cream cheese
4 ounces Sugar-Free Chocolate Chips from Lily
Two tsp of extract from vanilla beans
Two and a half cups heavy cream
One teaspoon of instant powdered coffee, dry
DIRECTIONS 1. Make Atkins Soy-Free Flour Mix according to the Atkins recipe; you'll
need 1/2 cup.
2. Turn the oven on to 425°F. After cutting a circle of parchment paper to fit into the
bottom of a 9-inch pie pan, oil the pie plate, then insert the parchment.
Regarding the crust: Pulse the 1/2 cup baking mix, 4 teaspoons cocoa powder, cinnamon,
and 3 tablespoons sugar substitute in a food processor for approximately 10 seconds to
blend. Add the cold, chopped butter and pulse for 30 seconds or until the mixture
resembles coarse grain. Add the cream cheese and pulse for a further 30 seconds or until
the mixture starts to come together.
3. Transfer dough to a 9-inch pie plate that has been prepped, and pat into an even layer
on the edges and bottom. Using a fork, prick the dough around fifteen times, then
decoratively crimp the edges. Bake for ten minutes, or until set, with a light cover of
aluminum foil on. Remove the lid and continue baking for an additional 8 to 10 minutes,
until the color turns light golden brown. Before filling, let the crust cool.

4.To make the filling, combine one teaspoon of vanilla extract with chocolate in medium-sized bowl. For about four minutes, over medium-high heat, cook one cup of
cream and instant coffee until they are almost boiling. After pouring over the chocolate
and waiting three minutes, stir to melt the chocolate. Fill pie shell, level top, and refrigerate for half an hour.
Beat the remaining cream, 4 tablespoons sugar substitute, 1 teaspoon vanilla extract, and
1 tablespoon cocoa powder in a medium bowl on high speed with an electric mixer until
medium peaks form, about 4 minutes. Cover with a coating of chocolate and freeze for a
minimum of 2.5 hours, or until solid.
 5. Take out of the freezer ten minutes prior to
serving

Atkins Sweet Potato-Pumpkin Purée 12.2gNet Carbs
Prep Time: 20 Minutes
Style:American
Cook Time: 80 Minutes
Phase: Phase 3
15 SERVINGS
2.7g
Protein
10.6g
Fat
2.5g
Fiber
159.3cal
Calories
INGREDIENTS
Three and a half big egg whites
18 3/4 ounces Pumpkin (Without Salt, Drained, Cooked, Boiled)
6 1/4 tablespoons Sucralose Based Sweetener (Sugar Substitute)
2/3 cup, half Pecan Nuts
2 pounds Sweet Potato
2/3 cup Heavy Cream

2/3 teaspoon Salt
2/3 teaspoon Pumpkin Pie Spice
2/3 teaspoon Cinnamon
1/3 cup Unsalted Butter Stick
DIRECTIONS
1.Heat oven to 250°F. Lightly butter a baking sheet.
2.Place egg whites in a medium mixing bowl; beat with an electric mixer at high speed
until foamy. Gradually add 3 tablespoons of sugar substitute and continue mixing just
until soft peaks formSpoon onto prepared baking sheet and spread with a spatula to
¼-inch thickness. Bake 35 minutes. Turn oven off; let meringue stand in oven for 45
minutes. 3.Crush meringue and place in a bowl. Add pecans and toss gently to combine.
Set aside.
4.While meringue is resting, place sweet potatoes in a medium saucepan. Cover with
water to 2 inches above potatoes and bring to a boil. Cook until tender, about 20 minutes,
and drain. Return saucepan to medium-high heat. Add potatoes, butter, cream, 2
tablespoons sugar substitute, salt, cinnamon, pumpkin pie spice and pumpkin puree.
5. Stir to combine. Mash with a potato masher until smooth. Heat through, about 1
minute.Transfer potato mixture to a serving dish and cover with meringue topping.

Atkins Vanilla-Coconut Ice Cream 6.9gNet Carbs
Prep Time: 240 Minutes
Style:American
Cook Time: 5 Minutes
Phase: Phase 2
8 SERVINGS *
5.3g
Protein
43.7g fat

2g
Fiber
435.8cal
Calories
INGREDIENTS
1 cup Dried Coconut
6 large Egg Yolks
3/4 cup Sucralose Based Sweetener (Sugar Substitute)
2 cups Heavy Cream
1 14 ounces can Coconut Cream
2 teaspoons Coconut Extract
1 teaspoon Vanilla Extract
1/4 teaspoon Salt
DIRECTIONS
One cup of desiccated coconut
Six big egg yolks
3/4 cup Sugar Substitute Sweetener Based on Sucralose
Two cups of heavy cream
One 14-oz can of coconut cream
Two tsp of coconut extract
One tsp vanilla extract
1/4 tsp salt
DIRECTIONS
1. Bake the coconut for five to seven minutes at 350°F, stirring once throughout that time.
Take out of the oven and put aside.
2. Whisk the yolks and sugar substitute together in a medium-sized bowl. Heat a medium-sized saucepan over medium-high heat and bring the heavy cream to a
simmer. While whisking continuously, slowly add one cup of cream into the yolk
mixture. Return the yolk mixture to the pot. We call this procedure tempering.
3. Cook over medium heat, stirring frequently, for about three to five minutes, or until
mixture is thick enough to coat the back of a spoon. Take off the heat. Add salt, coconut
milk, vanilla, and coconut extracts. Relax for four hours.
5. Fill the ice cream machine with the mixture. Follow the manufacturer's instructions for
processing. Add the toasted coconut five minutes before the ice cream is done.

Atkins Chocolate Chip-Macadamia Nut Ice Cream Sandwiches 6.8gNet Carbs

Prep Time: 300 Minutes

Style:American

Cook Time: 25 Minutes

Phase: Phase 2

10 SERVINGS

11g

Protein

47.1g

Fat

5g

Fiber

490.9cal

Calories

INGREDIENTS

1/2 cup Butter, salted

3/4 cup Sucralose Based Sweetener (Sugar Substitute)

2 teaspoons Vanilla Extract

3 large Eggs (Whole)

1 cup Atkins Flour Mix (cups)

1/2 teaspoon Baking powder

5 tablespoons Lily's Sugar Free Chocolate Chips

3 cups Heavy Cream

3 large Egg Yolks

1/4 teaspoon Salt

1/2 cup, whole or half Macadamia Nuts

1/2 teaspoon Pure Almond Extract

DIRECTIONS

1. Turn the oven on to 375°F.

One cup of Atkins Flour Mix is needed for the cookies. Smoothly blend 1/2 cup

granulated sugar replacement, 1 tsp vanilla, and melted butter. Once one egg has been

added, mix until smooth and thick. Blend in the baking powder and flour mixture until

smooth. Add the chocolate chips and fold. Divide the dough into twenty balls of the

same size. Place on a pan coated with parchment paper, space them 2 inches apart,
flatten a little, and bake for 10 to 12 minutes, or until gently browned. Put aside to cool.
2. For the ice cream with macadamia nuts: Transfer heavy cream into a 3-quart pot with a
heavy bottom and set it over medium heat. To prevent the cream from boiling over, bring
to a gentle boil and whisk often. Take off the heat.
3. Combine 2 eggs, 3 egg yolks, 1/4 cup sugar substitute, and salt in a large bowl. Beat
together with a whisk or a hand mixer until smooth and thickened.
To prevent curdling of the eggs, take about a cup of the hot cream from the pot using a
ladle and slowly whisk it into the egg mixture. Whisk the egg mixture and then pour it
into the saucepan with the remaining cream.
4.Switch for one to two minutes over medium heat, or until slightly thickened. Transfer
into a sanitized basin, stir in 1 tsp vanilla and almond extract, and let to stand for about
1.5 hours, or until custard has fully cooled to room temperature. Place in the refrigerator
for two hours or overnight, covered with plastic wrap.
5.Freeze in the ice cream machine as directed by the manufacturer. Frozen macadamia
nuts should be added 15 minutes before freezing is finished.
6. To put together sandwiches: Place ten cookies on the work surface, top side down. Working quickly, put 1/4 cup of ice cream on each cookie using an ice cream scoop.
Place another biscuit on top of each, bottom side down.
7. Thoroughly cover every sandwich in plastic wrap and store it in the freezer. For softer
ice cream, freeze for at least 4 hours, or overnight for firmer sandwiches. Keeps for up to
a month in the freezer.

CHAPTER 8: SMOOTHIES

Atkins Tropical Raspberry Smoothie11.4gNet Carbs
Prep Time: 5 Minutes
Style:Other
Cook Time: 0 Minutes
Phase: Phase 2
Difficulty: Moderate
3 SERVINGS
11.6g
Protein
29.7g
Fat
4.1g
Fiber
357.6cal
Calories
INGREDIENTS
1 1/2 cups Coconut Cream
12 ounces Firm Silken Tofu
1 1/2 cups Red Raspberries
6 teaspoons Sucralose Based Sweetener (Sugar Substitute)
1/2 teaspoon Coconut Extract
DIRECTIONS
1. In a blender, combine coconut milk, tofu, 1/2 cup raspberries, coconut extract, and
sugar substitute (if preferred); process until smooth. You may strain the mixture through a
sieve and then put it back in the blender if you want to get rid of the seeds.
2. Add three ice cubes at a time, one at a time, and mix until smooth while the machine is
operating.

3. Transfer into a large glass, and if like, top with raspberries and whipped cream. Serve
right away.
COOKING ADVICE
The serving options above may be updated to reflect the necessary quantity of ingredients, regardless of whether you're cooking for one person or a large family.

Atkins Banana-Coconut Rum Yummy10.7gNet Carbs
Prep Time: 5 Minutes
Style:Other
Cook Time: 0 Minutes
Phase: Phase 3
Difficulty: Moderate
1 SERVING *
2.3g
Protein
17.4g
Fat
0.9g
Fiber
264.2cal
Calories
COMPOSITION
one-third little (6" to 6-7/8" length) Banana
one-third cup coconut cream
One fluid ounce without ice Two ice cubes and rum Using Tap Water
One packet Stevia, or Truvia
DIRECTIONS
1.Use coconut rum or spiced rum to enhance the taste of this dish. Since most manufacturers do not include a nutritional label, make sure to check online to make sure
your flavored rum is free of added sugar. You may make this non-alcoholic by using half
a teaspoon of rum extract in place of the rum. Additionally, be sure to use canned
coconut milk or cream rather than sweetened coconut cream.
2. Fill a blender with the banana, canned coconut cream, rum, granular sugar replacement
(use 2 tsp and add 1 g NC to the total if using sucralose), and ice.

3. Blend on high until all of the ice is gone. Adapt the sweetener as
necessary.
4. Transfer into a martini glass and garnish with a sprinkling of cinnamon
or nutmeg, if
preferred.

Atkins Keto Avocado Gazpacho Smoothie 4.7gNet Carbs
Prep Time: 5 Minutes
Style:Mexican
Cook Time: 0 Minutes
Phase: Phase 1
Difficulty: Moderate
1 SERVING *
9.1g
Protein
38.2g
Fat
11.9g
Fiber
419.5cal
Calories
INGREDIENTS
1 fruit without skin and seed California Avocado
1 ounce Goat Cheese (Soft)
1 tablespoon Heavy Cream
2 teaspoons Fresh Lime Juice
1/8 teaspoon Salt
1 cup Tap Water
2 teaspoons chopped Chives
DIRECTIONS
1. Add the chopped avocado to a blender. Blend in the remaining
ingredients until
smooth. To get the right consistency, add a tablespoon at a time of
more water if
necessary.

2.. Transfer to a large glass, and if like, top with a saved avocado slice and chives. Serve
right away.

Atkins Vegan Almond-Raspberry Smoothie 8.3gNet Carbs
Prep Time: 5 Minutes
Style:American
Cook Time: 0 Minutes
Phase: Phase 2
Difficulty: Moderate
2 SERVINGS
30.5g
Protein
15.2g
Fat
7.5g
Fiber
300.8cal
Calories
COMPOSITION
1 and a third cups Original Pure Almond Milk, Unsweetened
Soy Protein Powder, two scoops
One cup of red raspberries
40 almonds each
DIRECTIONS
1. In a blender, mix together almond milk, raspberries, almonds, and one scoop (or the
equivalent of 25g protein; often 1 oz or 2 Tbsp) of protein powder until smooth. Blend in
two ice cubes, if desired.

Atkins Raspberry-Teani7.5gNet Carbs

Net Carbs

0.3g

Protein

0.1g

Fat

1.4g

Fiber

76.1cal

Calories

INGREDIENTS

1 tea bag Raspberry Zinger Herbal Tea

1 1/2 teaspoons Sweetener

1 fluid ounce (no ice) Vodka

10 each Red Raspberries

1 wedge or slice (1/8 of one 2-1/8" dia lemon) Lemon

DIRECTIONS This recipe may also be used to produce a delicious nonalcoholic spritzer
that is appropriate for Phase 1. Just pour 4 ounces of club soda in lieu of the vodka, then
serve over ice.

1. Prepare the non-caloric herbal raspberry tea. Steep in 1/2 cup boiling water for 5–6
minutes. Put the cup in an ice water bath for five to ten minutes to swiftly cool it.

Grind the granular sugar substitute (we suggest 2. Truvia brand sweetener) in a large
martini mixer. 9 raspberries (save 1 for garnish), vodka, and sucralose (use 4 tsp and add
2g NC per serving).

3. Include the ice, squeeze the lemon slice, and pour the cooled raspberry tea.

4. Shake well to mix, strain, and transfer into a chilled martini glass with a raspberry on
top.

COOKING ADVICE

Why not have this cocktail with some pals over? Change the serving options above to see
how much of each ingredient you'll need.

Atkins Almond-Pineapple Smoothie16.1gNet Carbs
Prep Time: 5 Minutes
Style:American
Cook Time: 0 Minutes
Phase: Phase 3
Difficulty: Moderate
3 SERVINGS
10.7g
Protein
17.3g
Fat
3.9g
Fiber
275.7cal
Calories
INGREDIENTS
1 1/2 cups (8 fluid ounces) Plain Yogurt (Whole Milk)
7 1/2 ounces Pineapple
60 each wholes Blanched & Slivered Almonds
1 1/2 cups Pure Almond Milk - Unsweetened Original
DIRECTIONS 1. Feel free to swap out the pineapple and/or almonds (about 20 whole
almonds, 3 Tbsp slivered) with other fruits or nuts. Make sure the pineapple in this
smoothie is fresh. Pineapple in a can has a lot of sugar.
In a blender, combine the yogurt, almond milk, pineapple, and almonds; process until
smooth and creamy.

CHAPTER 9: APPETIZERS

APPETIZER RECIPE 1

Atkins Keto Swiss Chard with Garlic Butter 2.7g
Net Carbs
Prep Time: 15 Minutes
Style:Other
Cook Time: 15 Minutes
Phase: Phase 1
Difficulty: Moderate
8 SERVINGS *
2.1g
Protein
4.9g
Fat
1.8g
Fiber
63.2cal
Calories
INGREDIENTS
2 pounds Swiss Chard
2 tablespoons Unsalted Butter Stick
1 tablespoon Light Olive Oil
2 teaspoons Garlic
1/2 teaspoon Salt
1/4 teaspoon Black Pepper

DIRECTIONS
1. Chop the stems of chard crosswise into 1/2-inch segments. Leaves should be cut in half
lengthwise, stacked, and then cut into 2-inch pieces crosswise.
2. In a large saucepan, melt the butter and olive oil over medium heat. Add the garlic and
stir-fry for approximately 30 seconds, or until it becomes aromatic. Add the chard stems;
cover and simmer for approximately 4 minutes, stirring periodically, until the stems are
crisp-tender.
3. Season with salt and pepper and add the chard leaves in batches, stirring to coat. For
four to five minutes, or until the stems are soft and the leaves have wilted, cover and
simmer, stirring once.

Atkins 3.3g of Tomato-Cucumber GuacamoleNet Carbs
15 minutes for preparation
Mexican fashion
Cooking Period: None
Phase: First Phase
Moderate in difficulty
Protein: * 8 Servings * 1.5g
6.8g of fat
3.8 grams of fiber
87.8 kcal of calories
COMPOSITION
Two entire medium (2–3/5" in diameter) crimson tomatoes
2 medium-sized peeled cucumbers
Two fruit void of seeds and skin Avocados from California
1/4 cup of finely chopped red onions
One and a half fluid ounces Juice from fresh limes
Half a teaspoon of cumin
DIRECTIONS
Cut the onions, cucumber, avocado, and tomatoes into dice. Zest and juice the lime.
Gently combine tomatoes, cucumbers, avocados, onion, 1 tsp lime zest, 3 Tbsp lime
juice, and cumin in a medium-sized bowl.
Add pepper and salt to taste.

Atkins Kale with Pears and Onions 11.1gNet Carbs
Prep Time: 15 Minutes
Style:American
Cook Time: 30 Minutes
Phase: Phase 3
6 SERVINGS *
2.8g
Protein
7.4g
Fat
2.7g
Fiber
122cal
Calories
INGREDIENTS
1 pound Kale
3 tablespoons Extra Virgin Olive Oil
1 medium (2-1/2" diameter) Onions
1 pear, medium (approx 2-1/2 per lb) Pears
1/4 teaspoon Curry Powder
1/8 teaspoon Nutmeg (Ground)
1/2 teaspoon Salt
1/4 teaspoon Black Pepper
DIRECTIONS
1. Cook the kale for approximately three minutes, or until it becomes brilliant green and
wilts, in a big saucepan of boiling, lightly salted water. Squeeze out excess liquid, drain,
let cool for ten minutes, then finely chop.
2. Put a big nonstick skillet over medium-high heat with oil. Add the onion slices and
simmer for 6 to 7 minutes, stirring now and again, until the onion is softly brown.
Add sliced pear and heat for 2 to 3 minutes, or until crisp-tender.
3. Add the curry and nutmeg, and simmer for 30 seconds or until aromatic.
Add the kale, salt, and pepper, and simmer for 3 to 4 minutes, turning regularly, or until
the kale is soft. Warm up and serve.

Atkins Ratatouille 5.9g7Net Carbs
Prep Time: 30 Minutes
Style:French
Cook Time: 45 Minutes
Phase: Phase 1
6 SERVINGS *
2.2g
Protein
12.3g
Fat
4.6g
Fiber
150.8cal
Calories
COMPOSITION
One unpeeled eggplant (about 1.4 lbs.) eggplant
One-third cup of extra virgin olive oil
two tsp of garlic
One medium zucchini
One tsp salt
Half a teaspoon of dried rosemary
Half a tablespoon of dried thyme leaves
One little onion and 1/4 teaspoon of black pepper
One tiny whole sweet red pepper, about 2-2/5" in diameter crimson
tomato
Merely one medium yellow summer squash
DIRECTIONS
1. After lightly salting the eggplant, put it in a sieve and let the bitter juices
to drain for
20 minutes. After rinsing, gently dry the eggplant.
Preheat the oven to 425°F. Combine oil, minced garlic, salt, rosemary,
thyme, and pepper
in a 10 x 15 baking dish. Dice all the veggies, including the eggplant, evenly,
and then
combine them with the oil mixture in the baking dish.
3. Bake the dish for 15 minutes with the foil covering it. After 30 minutes of
cooking,
uncover and stir periodically, until the veggies are soft and caramelized.

Atkins Broccoli Rabe Parmigiano1.7gNet Carbs
Prep Time: 15 Minutes
Style:Italian
Cook Time: 10 Minutes
Phase: Phase 1
Difficulty: Moderate
6 SERVINGS *
8.1g
Protein
7.6g
Fat
3.9g
Fiber
112.4cal
Calories
INGREDIENTS
Two Tbsp. Pure Virgin Olive Oil
two garlic cloves
Crushed red pepper flakes, 1/4 teaspoon
Fresh broccoli rabe, two pounds
one-fourth cup of tap water
two tsp Fresh Lemon Juice
two tsp Zest of Lemon
1/8 teaspoon of salt
one-eighth teaspoon of black pepper
Half a cup of grated Parmesan cheese
DIRECTIONS
1. Broccoli rabe has scattered clusters of small broccoli-like buds on 6- to 9-inch stems. It
tastes bitterer than its more recognizable relative. It makes a delicious sauté or braising. If
you'd like, you can definitely make this dish without the broccoli. Peel and chop the
stems of a 2-pound head of broccoli into 1/2-inch pieces after cutting it into tiny florets.
2. Heat the oil in a big, deep skillet over medium-high heat. Add the pepper flakes and
minced garlic, and sauté for 30 seconds.
3. Mix well after adding the broccoli rabe, water, and lemon juice. Broccoli rabe should
be crisp-tender after 8 minutes of cooking in a covered pan over medium heat.

Add salt and freshly ground black pepper to taste.
Transfer to a platter, then top with Parmesan cheese.
Atkins Tabbouleh Salad12gNet Carbs
Prep Time: 25 Minutes
Style:American
Cook Time: 0 Minutes
Phase: Phase 3
Difficulty: Difficult
6 SERVINGS *
2.8g
Protein
9.3g
Fat
3.9g
Fiber
149.5cal
Calories
INGREDIENTS
One parsley
Eight tsp peppermint (mint)
Three huge spring onions, or scallions
One-fourth cup of extra virgin olive oil
one-fourth cup of freshly squeezed lemon juice
One tsp salt
Half a teaspoon of black pepper
DIRECTIONS
In a large heatproof dish, combine bulgur and water. Tightly cover with plastic wrap and
let stand until water is absorbed, approximately 15 minutes.
To get rid of extra water, put bulgur in a sieve lined with cheesecloth or dishtowel and
push down hard with your hands.

toss gently to incorporate with tomatoes, cucumber, parsley, mint, oil, lemon juice,
scallions, salt, and pepper. Refrigerate or serve room temperature.

APPETIZER 2

Atkins Wild Rice, Sausage and Cherry Stuffing 9.2gNet Carbs

Prep Time: 60 Minutes

Style:American

Cook Time: 45 Minutes

Phase: Phase 3

Difficulty: Difficult

8 SERVINGS *

11.3g

Protein

16.6g

Fat

1.7g

Fiber

235.1cal

Calories

INGREDIENTS

3/4 cup chopped Onions

4 servings Atkins Low Carb Wheat Bread

1/3 cup Wild Rice

2 1/2 cups Tap Water

12 ounce raw (yield after cooking) Italian Sausage

1/4 cup Unsalted Butter Stick

3 stalk, medium (7-1/2" - 8" long) Celery

1/2 cup Parsley

1/3 cup, with pits, yield Red Sour Cherries

1 tablespoon Poultry Seasoning

1/2 teaspoon Black Pepper

1 cup Chicken Broth, Bouillon or Consomme

DIRECTIONS

To prepare Atkins Cuisine Bread, follow the Atkins recipe.

1. In a small saucepan, combine the wild rice, 1 1/2 cups water, and a big amount of salt.

Over high heat, bring to a boil. Simmer for 40 to 45 minutes on low heat with a lid on

until the food is soft.

2. Empty and reserve.

Preheat the oven to 350°F. Arrange the bread cubes in a single layer on a jelly-roll pan.

Bake for 10 to 14 minutes, stirring once, or until crispy. Move to a big bowl

3. Meanwhile, take off the sausage from its casing and crumble it into a big nonstick pan
that you heat to medium. Simmer for about 12 minutes, turning often to break up any
clumps, or until cooked through and gently browned. Mix with bread.
4. Put the skillet back on medium heat and add the butter. After butter has melted, add the
white onion and celery and simmer, stirring often, until it becomes soft, approximately 10
minutes.
5.Add to bread mixture, then stir in parsley, cherries, poultry seasoning, pepper and wild
rice. Blend well. Add more chicken broth if the stuffing seems dry after mixing in one
cup.
6. Spoon the filling into a large baking dish. Cover with foil and bake 30 minutes, then
uncover and continue baking until lightly browned and heated through, 15 minutes
longer.

Atkins Keto Mushroom Salad with Walnuts and Watercress 2.9g
Net Carbs
Prep Time: 15 Minutes
Style:American
Cook Time: 16 Minutes
Phase: Phase 2
Difficulty: Difficult
4 SERVINGS *
4g
Protein
17.1g
Fat
1.4g
Fiber
176.4cal
Calories

INGREDIENTS
1 1/2 ounces English Walnuts
2 tablespoons chopped Shallots
1/4 teaspoon Salt
1 tablespoon Red Wine Vinegar
3 tablespoons Extra Virgin Olive Oil
2 caps Portobello Mushroom Cap
4 cups chopped Watercress
DIRECTIONS
1. Because it contains nuts, this dish is appropriate for all phases of the Atkins diet, with
the exception of the first two weeks of Induction.
2. Turn the oven on to 350°F. After toasting for 7–8 minutes, take the walnuts out of the
oven, let them cool, and then cut.
3. Set the oven to broil.
In a bowl, mix shallot, vinegar, and salt for the vinaigrette. Add two tablespoons of oil
and whisk to combine. Add pepper to taste.
4. Apply the remaining oil to the mushrooms and season with salt and pepper. For 4
minutes on each side, grill or broil 4 from the heat source. Slice the mushrooms into long,
thin pieces. Add a spoonful of vinaigrette and toss.
5. Spoon the remaining vinaigrette equally over each salad dish after arranging the
watercress and walnuts. Place the mushrooms on top.

Atkins Atkins Cornbread2.3gNet Carbs
Prep Time: 10 Minutes
Style:American
Cook Time: 30 Minutes
Phase: Phase 3
16 SERVINGS *
8.6g
Protein
12.7g
Fat

12.7g
Fat
0.5g
Fiber
154.4cal
Calories
INGREDIENTS
3 large Eggs
1 cup Whole Milk
1/3 cup Vegetable Oil
2 tablespoons Unsalted Butter Stick
8 ounces Monterey Jack Cheese with Jalapeno
1 each Chipotle en Adobo, whole
1/2 cup Whole Grain Soy Flour
2 ounces Vital Wheat Gluten
3 teaspoons Baking Powder (Sodium Aluminum Sulfate, Double Acting)
DIRECTIONS
Set oven temperature to 350°F.
Use olive oil spray to lightly coat an 8-inch square baking pan.
2. Beat the egg, milk, oil, and melted butter in a medium-sized basin. Add the chopped
chiles and shredded cheeses, and toss until well combined.
3. Add the baking powder, soy flour, and 1/4 cup of wheat gluten. Stir just until the
ingredients are incorporated; the mixture will be stiff. Fill prepared pan with mixture.
Bake till the color becomes golden.
4. Let cool for five to ten minutes on a wire rack before slicing into sixteen 2-by-2-inch
squares for serving.

Atkins Keto Herb-Butter Blend 0.1net carb
Prep Time: 7 Minutes
Style:American
Cook Time: 0 Minutes
Phase: Phase 1
Difficulty: Moderate
32 SERVINGS *
0.1g
Protein
12.5g
Fat
0.1g
Fiber
110.7cal
Calories
INGREDIENTS
1/2 teaspoon Salt
1 teaspoon Black Pepper
1/2 cup Extra Virgin Olive Oil
1 teaspoon Garlic
3 teaspoons leaves Oregano
2 tablespoons Basil
1 cup Unsalted Butter Stick
1/2 cup Coconut Oil
DIRECTIONS
1. Meats, seafood, and veggies all taste great with this flavorful butter. One tablespoon is
given each.
2. Fill a food processor with salt, pepper, olive oil, garlic, oregano, and basil. Pulse for 30
to 60 seconds, or until herbs are finely crushed and pepper flecks are not visible.
3. Blend in coconut oil and butter until smooth.
Scrape into a snap-top jar and store in the refrigerator for up to one month.

Atkins Keto Egg Drop Soup1.5gNet Carbs
Prep Time: 5 Minutes
Style:Asian
Cook Time: 10 Minutes
Phase: Phase 1
Difficulty: Moderate
4 SERVINGS *
7.7g
Protein
4.3g
Fat
0.2g
Fiber
79.4cal
Calories
COMPOSITION
Two 14.5-oz cans of Bouillon, Consomme, or Chicken Broth
One tsp of ginger
Two huge (whole) eggs
Two medium-sized (4-1/8-inch long) spring onions or scallops
One-half tsp toasted sesame oil
DIRECTIONS
1. Bring the broth and minced ginger to a boil in a medium saucepan over high heat. 2.
Lower the heat to a simmer and gradually add the egg to create golden threads.
2.After turning off the heat, add the soy sauce, sesame oil, and chopped green onions to
taste. Serve right away.
COOKING ADVICE
Instead of ordering takeout, try this naturally low-carb and ketogenic homemade egg drop
soup with our recipe for Asian Veggie and Pork Bowl.

VEGETARIAN RECIPES: CHAPTER 10

Atkins Vegetarian "Sausage" Sauté with Red Bell Pepper and
Onions6.9g
Net Carbs
Prep Time: Minutes
Style:American
Cook Time: 0 Minutes
Phase: Phase 1
Difficulty: Moderate
1 SERVING *
27.4g
Protein
28.9g
Fat
2.7g
Fiber
406.4cal
Calories
INGREDIENTS
1/8 cup chopped Red Sweet Pepper
1 tablespoon Extra Virgin Olive Oil
1/4 cup shredded Cheddar Cheese
2 tablespoons chopped Onions
2 patties Veggie Breakfast Sausage Patties
DIRECTIONS
1. Saute white onion and red bell peppers in olive oil in a pan
over medium heat until
tender.
2. Add the crushed sausage patties and stir periodically while
cooking until browned.
3.Add cheese on top, then serve right away.

Atkins Keto Scrambled Eggs with Goat Cheese and Asparagus2.2g
Net Carbs
Prep Time: 5 Minutes
Style:American
Cook Time: 5 Minutes
Phase: Phase 1
Difficulty: Moderate
1 SERVING *
22.3g
Protein
24.6g
Fat
1g
Fiber
324.5cal
Calories
COMPOSITION
Three medium spears (5-1/4" to 7" long) asparagus
One tsp olive oil
Two big eggs, entire
One ounce of firm goat cheese
GUIDELINES
1. Put a small nonstick pan over medium-high heat with two tablespoons of water. When
the water has evaporated and the asparagus is tender, add it and steam. 2. Take out the
asparagus and reheat.
3. Heat a pan with a teaspoon of virgin olive oil over medium heat. Add the eggs and goat
cheese, and scramble until the cheese is melted and the eggs are set.
4. Add the asparagus on top. Serve right away after adding salt and freshly ground black
pepper to taste.

Atkins Vegetarian "Turkey" and Provolone Cheese Roll-Ups8.2g

Net Carbs

Prep Time: 5 Minutes

Style:American

Cook Time: 0 Minutes

Phase: Phase 2

Difficulty: Moderate

2 SERVINGS

66.2g

Protein

63.9g

Fat

8.9g

Fiber

891.5cal

Calories

COMPOSITION

three portions Cunning Deli Roast Turkey Method

Two tsp Dijon Mustard

One fruit (seed and skin removed) Avocado from California

Twelve ounces Provolone Cheese

DIRECTIONS

Apply mustard on both "turkey" slices.

After adding cheese, wrap up.

Atkins Lettuce-Wrapped Cheddar Veggie Burger with Avocado and Onion 3.1g

Net Carbs

Prep Time: 5 Minutes

Style:American

Cook Time: 10 Minutes

Phase: Phase 1

Difficulty: Moderate

2 SERVING *
24.1g
Protein
29.2g
Fat
12.3g
Fiber
394.2cal
Calories
INGREDIENTS
1 burger All American Classic Meatless Burgers
1 teaspoon Extra Virgin Olive Oil
1 tablespoon chopped Onions
1 slice (1 ounce) Cheddar Cheese
1/2 fruit without skin and seed California Avocados
3 leaves Butterhead Lettuce (Includes Boston and Bibb Types)
DIRECTIONS
Cook the veggie burger with 1 tsp oil in a pan over medium-high heat or in the
microwave. Warm up fully. White onions may be sautéed in the same pan as the veggie
burger.
Add cheese, onions, and avocado slices on top.

Encase in lettuce. Have fun!
Atkins Eggplant Rollatini11.6gNet Carbs
Prep Time: 20 Minutes
Style:Italian
Cook Time: 75 Minutes
6 SERVINGS *
26.6g
Protein
32.1g
Fat
6.2g
Fiber
456.3cal
Calories

INGREDIENTS
24 ounces Eggplant
1 1/2 cups Tap Water
3/4 cup Whole Grain Soy Flour
4 large Eggs (Whole)
1/4 cup Extra Virgin Olive Oil
1 1/4 cups Tomato Sauce (Canned)
2 cups Ricotta Cheese (Whole Milk)
4 ounces Mozzarella Cheese, whole milk
1/3 cup Parmesan Cheese (Grated)
1/4 cup Parsley
1/4 teaspoon Salt
1/4 teaspoon Black Pepper
DIRECTIONS
1. Cut eggplants into 1/8- to 1/4-inch slices, then place them in a colander, gently salting
each layer. After allowing the bitter juices to drip for fifteen minutes, rinse and pat dry.
2. In a large bowl, blend two eggs, soy flour, and water until smooth. In a heavy, big pan,
heat approximately ¼ cup olive oil over medium-high heat until heated but not smoking.
3. Add the eggplant to the pan after dipping each slice in the batter. Cook eggplant in batches for 2 to 3 minutes, stirring regularly, until soft and golden (slices should not touch). As needed, add more oil. After draining, place the eggplant slices on paper towels
and chill them on a wire rack.
4. Preheat the oven to 400 degrees Fahrenheit. Grease a 13x9 baking dish very lightly.
Pour half a cup of tomato sauce into the pan and tilt it to cover the bottom.
5. To make the filling, combine the ricotta, mozzarella, leftover eggs, Parmesan cheese,
parsley, salt, and pepper in a big basin. Using a wooden spoon, stir everything together
until thoroughly combined.
6. To make rollatini, center an eggplant slice with a heaping spoonful of filling, then roll
it up. Repeat to make 24 rolls. Arrange the rolls in rows in the prepared pan, seam side
down. Transfer the leftover tomato sauce over the rolls' tops. Tightly cover pan with foil.
Bake for 30 minutes, then take off the foil and bake for a further 10 minutes, or until bubbling and just beginning to brown.

CHAPTER 11:LOW CARB VEGAN RECIPE

Vegan recipe 1
Peanut-Tofu Cabbage Wraps
Cook Time:30 mins
Total Time:
30 mins
Servings:
4
Yield:
4 servings
Nutrition Profile:
Low-Carb Dairy-Free Low Added Sugar Vegan Vegetarian Egg-Free
Gluten-Free
Low-Calorie
INGREDIENTS
8 small napa or Savoy cabbage leaves or 4 large, cut in half crosswise
1 tablespoon canola oil
1 14- to 16-ounce package extra-firm tofu, patted dry and crumbled
¼ teaspoon salt
5 tablespoons prepared peanut sauce
1 tablespoon rice vinegar
1 ½ teaspoons lime zest
1 cup julienned Asian pear
1 cup julienned English cucumber
¼ cup finely chopped cilantro
DIRECTIONS
1. Thoroughly wash and pat dry the cabbage leaves, then remove any
tough stems or ribs.
2. Put a big nonstick skillet over medium-high heat with oil. Add the
tofu, season with
salt, and cook for 4 to 6 minutes, turning often, or until it is barely
golden brown.
3. In the meanwhile, combine lime zest, vinegar, and peanut sauce in a
small dish.

4. Take the pan off of the burner, pour in the sauce mixture, and mix everything together.

Present the tofu enclosed in cabbage leaves, garnished with cucumber, pear, and cilantro.

Nutrition Facts

(per serving)

186

Calories

12g

Fat

8g

Carbs

13g

Protein

Vegan Burrito Bowls with Cauliflower Rice

Prep Time:

25 mins

Total Time:

25 mins

Servings:

4

Yield:

4 containers

INGREDIENTS

1 recipe Tofu Crumbles

1 (12 ounce) package frozen riced cauliflower

4 teaspoons olive oil

1 teaspoon no-salt-added taco seasoning

1 cup thinly sliced red cabbage

1 cup diced avocado

½ cup pico de gallo or salsa

¼ cup chopped fresh cilantro

PREPARE TOFU CRUMBLES AS DIRECTED.

1. Prepare the riced cauliflower per the instructions on the box while the tofu crumbles

simmer. Add oil and taco spice and toss.

2. Distribute the cauliflower among four lidded single-serving containers. Add 1/4 cup of
each of the cabbage and avocado, 1/2 cup of beefless ground beef, 2 teaspoons of pico de
gallo (or salsa), and 1 tablespoon of cilantro on top of each. When you're ready to eat,
seal the containers and keep them chilled.
Nutrition Information (per serving)
298 energy
15g Carbs and 20g Fat
15 grams of protein
Mushroom & Tofu Stir-Fry
Prep Time:
20 mins
Total Time:
20 mins
Servings:
5
Yield:
5 servings
COMPOSITION
One pound of mixed mushrooms, one medium red bell pepper, one bunch of chopped
onions, and four tablespoons of peanut or canola oil, split into two-inch chunks.
One tablespoon of freshly grated ginger
One big clove of grated garlic; one 8-ounce package of baked or smoked tofu; three
tablespoons of chopped oyster sauce; or vegetarian oyster sauce (see Tip)
DIRECTIONS
1. In a large cast-iron pan or wok with a flat bottom, heat 2 tablespoons oil over high
heat. Add the bell pepper and mushrooms and simmer, stirring often, until softened,
approximately 4 minutes. Add the garlic, ginger, and scallions and heat for an additional
30 seconds. Place the veggies in a bowl.
2. Add the tofu and the last two teaspoons of oil to the pan. Cook for 3 to 4 minutes,
flipping once, or until browned. Add the oyster sauce and veggies and stir. Stir and heat
for about one minute.

Advice: Oysters, salt, sugar, and sometimes soy sauce are the main ingredients of sweet,
salty oyster sauce. If you want, you may use a vegetarian stir-fry sauce or oyster sauce
that utilizes mushrooms in place of oysters.

Nutrition Facts
(per serving)

171
Calories

13g
Fat

9g
Carbs

8g
Protein

Thai Coconut Curry Soup

Prep Time:
50 mins

Total Time:
50 mins

Servings:
8

Yield:
8 serving

INGREDIENTS

Six cups low-sodium vegetable broth, divided ¾ ounce dried shiitake mushrooms

A solitary spoonful of unadulterated olive oil

half a cup of finely chopped onion

two tsp of fresh ginger, coarsely chopped

Two jalapeño peppers, minced

One and a half tablespoons Thai red curry pasteHalf a teaspoon of low-sodium tamari

½ teaspoon salt, 1/2 cup lime juice, and 1/4 teaspoon lime zest

one and a half cups coconut milk

Twelve ounces of finely diced, extra-firm tofu (1/2-inch)

Three ounces of recently chopped wild mushrooms, such as oyster

Add the dried shiitake mushrooms to one cup of broth in a small saucepan. Turn the heat
up to medium-high and bring to a boil. For ten minutes, cook with a lid on and reduced
heat to maintain a simmer. Press the mushrooms to extract as much liquid as possible
after straining the broth through a second layer of cheesecloth or a coffee filter to get rid
of any grit. Chop the mushrooms and save aside the liquid used for cooking.
In the meanwhile, warm up some oil in a big saucepan over medium-high heat. Add the
onion and simmer for 2 to 4 minutes, stirring often, or until it begins to brown. Reduce
the heat to medium and simmer, stirring often, until the onion is soft, 3 to 5 minutes.
Scrape up any browned pieces and stir in the remaining 5 cups of liquid. Over high heat,
cover and bring to a boil. Add the saved mushroom-cooking liquid, ginger, jalapeños,
curry paste, tamari, lime zest and juice, and salt. Bring back to a boil, covered.
Lower the heat to medium and include the tofu, coconut milk, fresh mushrooms, and
soaked shiitakes. Simmer and partly cover until the mushrooms become soft, which
should take around three to five minutes. Add the spinach and simmer for a further two to
three minutes, or until it wilts. If preferred, top with cilantro and serve.

Chipotle-Orange Broccoli & Tofu
Cook Time:
30 mins
Total Time:
30 mins
Servings:
4
Yield:
4 servings, about 1 1/ cups each
INGREDIENTS
1 14-ounce package extra-firm water-packed tofu
½ teaspoon salt, divided
3 tablespoons canola oil, divided
6 cups broccoli florets
1 cup orange juice
1 tablespoon minced chipotle in adobo (see Tip), seeded if desired
½ cup chopped fresh cilantro

DIRECTIONS 3. After draining and patting dry, chop the tofu into 1/2- to 3/4-inch cubes.
Season the tofu with 1/4 teaspoon salt on both sides. In a large nonstick pan set over
medium-high heat, heat 2 tablespoons of oil. Add the tofu and cook it in a single layer for
7 to 9 minutes, stirring every few minutes, or until it becomes golden brown. Move to a
platter.
2. Add the remaining 1 tablespoon oil to the pan, along with the broccoli and the remaining 1/4 teaspoon salt. Cook, stirring, for 1 minute or until the broccoli is brilliant
green. Stir the broccoli often for another two to three minutes, or until it is just tender,
after adding the orange juice and chipotle.
Put the tofu back in the pan. Cook for one to two minutes, stirring gently, or until the tofu
is well cooked. Take off the heat and add the cilantro.

Raw Vegan Zoodles With Romesco
Prep Time:
20 mins
Total Time:
20 mins
Servings:
4
Yield:
5 cups
Nutrition Profile:
Low-Carb Diabetes-Appropriate Dairy-Free Healthy Immunity Low-Sodium Soy-Free
Heart-Healthy Vegan Vegetarian Egg-Free Gluten-Free Low-Calorie
INGREDIENTS
8 cups of medium-sized zucchini noodles
½ cup raw almonds; ½ teaspoon powdered pepper; ½ teaspoon divided salt
One medium red bell pepper, diced
Two teaspoons of extra virgin olive oil, cold-pressed
smashed little garlic cloves
One tsp of paprika
1/4 teaspoon of crushed red pepper and 1/4 teaspoon of ground cumin (optional)
DIRECTIONS
In a large bowl, toss zucchini noodles with 1/4 teaspoon each of salt and pepper.

In a small food processor, pulse almonds until they are finely chopped. Process the remaining 1/4 teaspoon salt, the red pepper, oil, garlic, paprika, cumin, crushed red pepper (if using), and red pepper until it becomes pretty smooth. Toss the zucchini with

3/4 of the red pepper sauce to coat. If preferred, sprinkle with a little more sauce and

serve.

Nutrition Information (per serving)

155 Calories

12g Fat, 9g Carbs

4 grams of protein

Easy Eggplant Stir-Fry

Active Time:

15 mins

Total Time:

15 mins

Servings:

6

Yield:

6 servings

Nutrition Profile:

Low-Sodium, Low-Carb, Dairy-Free, Vegan, Vegetarian, and Egg-Free

Which Eggplant Makes the Greatest Stir-Fries?

Any kind of eggplant can work in a stir-fry, but for this dish, we like Japanese eggplants

best. This kind of eggplant, also known as Asian or Chinese eggplant, is typically long

and thin with delicate purple skin and delicious, meaty flesh. They have a beautiful, solid

texture and a less bitter taste than rounder kinds because they contain fewer seeds. Farmers markets, Asian grocery shops, and well-stocked supermarkets are good places to

get Japanese eggplants. Mid- to late-summer is the best time to locate them. In the event

that Japanese eggplant is unavailable, a standard globe-shaped eggplant will suffice. To

make the eggplant stand up better while cooking, just chop it into smaller 1-inch pieces.

How to Perfectly Stir-Fry Eggplant

A nice sear on the exterior and soft, velvety flesh on the inside are the keys to well cooked eggplant. Instead of putting the whole eggplant in the pan at once, we do this by

frying it in stages. This added step permits instantaneous pan. This additional step adds

flavor and keeps the eggplant slices from coming apart by allowing the eggplant to brown

rather than steam. To keep warm while the second batch cooks, just move the first batch

to a bowl and cover it. Once the second batch is done, combine it with the first, then add
the other ingredients and mix with the sauce. And so it is! Perfect stir-fried eggplant.
COMPOSITION
4 Japanese eggplants (about 1 1/2 pounds)
Five tablespoons of peanut or canola oil, divided
2 tablespoons hoisin sauce
2 tablespoons reduced-sodium soy sauce
1 tablespoon plum sauce
2 jalapeño peppers, cut into thin rings
1 small yellow onion, sliced into 1/4-inch wedges
2 teaspoons minced garlic
1 teaspoon minced fresh ginger
1 cup packed fresh basil leaves
DIRECTIONS
Cut eggplants into quarters lengthwise, then into 2-inch pieces. Heat 2 tablespoons oil in
a large cast-iron skillet over high heat. Add half of the eggplant and cook, stirring occasionally, until tender and browned in parts, 4 to 5 minutes. Transfer to a large bowl.
Repeat with 2 tablespoons oil and the remaining eggplant. Cover the eggplant to keep
warm and set aside.
Meanwhile, whisk hoisin, soy sauce and plum sauce in a small bowl. Set aside.
Heat the remaining 1 tablespoon oil in the skillet over high heat. Add jalapeños and
onion; cook, stirring often, until slightly softened, 4 to 5 minutes. Add garlic and ginger;
cook, stirring often, until softened and fragrant, 30 seconds to 1 minute. Add the onion
mixture and basil to the eggplant and stir in the sauce. Serve immediately.
Nutrition Facts
(per serving)
161
Calories
12g
Fat
13g
Carbs
2g
Protein

VEGAN RECIPE 2

Slow-Cooker Curried Butternut Squash Soup
Prep Time:
10 mins
Additional Time:
3 hrs 35 mins
Total Time:
3 hrs 45 mins
Servings:8
INGREDIENTS
1 medium butternut squash (2-2 1/2 pounds), peeled, seeded and cubed (about 5 cups)
3 cups "no-chicken" broth or vegetable broth
1 medium onion, chopped
4 teaspoons curry powder
½ teaspoon garlic powder
¾ teaspoon salt
1 (14 ounce) can coconut milk
1-2 tablespoons lime juice, plus
wedges for serving
Chopped fresh cilantro for garnish
Nutrition Facts
(per serving)
153
Calories
11g
Fat
15g
Carbs
2g
Protein

Savory Orange-Roasted Tofu & Asparagus

Cook Time:

25 mins

Additional Time:

15 mins

Total Time:

40 mins

Servings:

4

Yield:

4 servings, scant 1 cup each

Nutrition Profile:

Low-Carb High-Calcium Bone-Health Healthy Aging Low Added Sugar Vegan Vegetarian Low-Calorie

INGREDIENTS

1 14-ounce package extra-firm water-packed tofu, rinsed

2 tablespoons red miso, (see Ingredient Note), divided

2 tablespoons balsamic vinegar, divided

4 teaspoons extra-virgin olive oil, divided

1 pound asparagus, trimmed and cut into 1-inch pieces

3 tablespoons chopped fresh basil

1 teaspoon freshly grated orange zest

¼ cup orange juice

¼ teaspoon salt

DIRECTIONS

Set oven temperature to 450°F. Apply cooking spray on a large baking sheet.

After drying off, cut the tofu into 1/2-inch pieces. In a large bowl, whisk together 1 tablespoon miso, 1 tablespoon vinegar, and 2 tablespoons oil until smooth. Toss gently to

coat after adding the tofu. On the baking sheet that has been prepared, evenly distribute

the tofu. Allow to roast for fifteen minutes. Toss asparagus gently with tofu. Go back to

the oven and continue roasting for an additional 8 to 10 minutes, or until the asparagus is

soft and the tofu is golden brown.In the meanwhile, use a large bowl to whisk together

the remaining 1 tablespoon miso, 1 tablespoon vinegar, 2 tablespoons oil, basil, orange

zest, and juice, and salt until they are smooth. Serve the roasted tofu and asparagus after

tossing them with the sauce.

Advice
A salty fermented paste prepared from barley, rice, and soybeans is called red miso
(akamiso). Locate it next to the tofu in the chilled department. Use it to make soups,
marinades, and sauces.
Simple cleanup: Cooking spray recipes may leave behind a sticky residue that is difficult
to remove. Before you spray the baking sheet with cooking spray, line it with a piece of
foil to save time and maintain its fresh appearance.
Nutrition Information (per serving)
154 Calories
11g Carbs and 9g Fat
10 grams of protein

Greenb Curry Soup
Cook Time:
1 hr 15 mins
Total Time:
1 hr 15 mins
Servings:
5
Yield:
6 servings, about 1 2/3 cups each
Nutrition Profile:
Low-Carb Healthy Immunity Low Added Sugar Vegan Vegetarian Gluten-Free Low-Calorie
COMPOSITION
Two medium-sized yellow onions
Divide the ½ teaspoon salt, 2 tablespoons + 2 teaspoons extra-virgin olive oil, and 2
tablespoons Thai green curry paste (see Note).
Five cups of homemade or store-bought vegetable broth
8 cups of gently packed spinach (approximately 6 ounces), split into 2 cups of water, and
any rough stems cut
One and a half cups of chopped oyster or shiitake mushrooms (approximately 4 ounces),
two big cloves of garlic, and trimmed 1 inch trimmed green bean bits
One cup of peeled and finely cut broccoli stems
Five scallions, cut into slices

1 tablespoon of lemongrass, chopped finely (see Note)one cup of freshly chopped
cilantro
One freshly chopped serrano chile and two tablespoons of fresh lemon juice, or
more to
taste.

DIRECTIONS

Slice onions thinly crosswise after quartering them lengthwise. In a soup pot or
Dutch
oven, heat 2 tablespoons of oil over medium-high heat. Add the onions and 1/4
teaspoon
of salt. Cook, stirring regularly, for 6 to 8 minutes, or until the onions are tender
and
starting to brown. Add the green curry paste and simmer for three minutes while
stirring.
Add 4 cups of broth and stir; reduce heat to a simmer.
In the meanwhile, roughly chop 4 cups of spinach. In a blender, add the remaining
4 cups
spinach and water; purée until the spinach resembles tiny pieces of confetti. Slice
the
mushrooms thinly, about 1/4 inch.
In a large pan, heat the remaining 2 tablespoons of oil over medium heat. Add the
garlic
and stir-fry for approximately 30 seconds, or until fragrant. Add the mushrooms
and
simmer, stirring, for 4 to 6 minutes, or until the liquid evaporates and the
mushrooms start
to take on color.
Add the green beans and mushroom combination to the saucepan, cover, and boil
for an
additional five minutes. Add the lemongrass, scallions, and broccoli stems.
Simmer for an
additional three minutes. Add the chopped and pureed spinach, chopped
cilantro, and a
generous amount of serrano pepper. Put the pot back on a simmer, cover it, and
cook the
spinach for about a minute, just enough to wilt it. If you would want a thinner
consistency, add up to 1 cup more broth. Juice from the lemon is added. Taste,
then adjust
with extra salt, serrano, or juice, if preferred.

Nutrition Information (per serving)
118 Calories
13g Carbs, 7g Fat,
and 3g Protein

Marinated Tofu Salad
Active Time:
25 mins
Total Time:
55 mins
Servings:
4
Nutrition Profile:
Low-Carb Dairy-Free Vegan Vegetarian Egg-Free Gluten-Free
INGREDIENTS
2 tablespoons extra-virgin olive oil
3 tablespoons fresh lemon juice
1 teaspoon ground cumin
1 teaspoon ground coriander
¾ teaspoon salt
1 (14 ounce) package extra-firm tofu, patted dry and cubed (3/4-inch)
2 tablespoons tahini
4 cups chopped romaine lettuce
2 cups peeled, seeded and chopped cucumber
2 medium plum tomatoes, seeded and chopped
½ cup finely chopped red onion
DIRECTIONS
In a big zip-top plastic bag, combine oil, lemon juice, garlic, cumin, coriander, and salt.
Add the tofu, close the bag, and give it a little shake to mix. For a minimum of 30
minutes and a maximum of 2 hours, refrigerate.
A big nonstick skillet should be heated over medium-high heat. Using a slotted spoon,
remove the tofu from the marinade; keep the marinade in the bag. Cook for 4 to 5
minutes, or until the bottom of the tofu is browned. In 4 to 5 minutes, flip and continue
cooking until the other side is browned.
Transfer the marinade that was set aside to a big bowl. Whisk in the tahini to blend it in.
Toss to coat and add the lettuce, cucumber, tomatoes, and onion. Place the heated tofu on
top of the salad.
Nutrition Information (per serving)
331 Calories

13g Carbs and 26g Fat
13 g of protein

Toasted Walnuts with a Winter Salad
Twenty minutes for preparation
Total Time:
20 mins
Servings:
4
Yield:
4 servings, 2 cups each
Ingredients Walnut Dressing
1 medium shallot, finely diced
1 tablespoon red-wine vinegar
1 teaspoon Dijon mustard
Half a teaspoon of salt
¼ cup walnut oil
Salad
4 cups mixed salad greens, such as watercress, Boston, escarole and/or curly endive, torn
into bite-size pieces
1 Belgian endive, cut crosswise into thin slices
1 small fennel bulb, trimmed and cut into 2-inch slivers
4 ounces white mushrooms, sliced
¼ cup chopped walnuts, toasted
Directions
To prepare vinaigrette: Combine shallot, vinegar, mustard and salt in a small bowl. Let
stand for 5 minutes, then whisk in oil.
To prepare salad: Combine salad greens, endive, fennel and mushrooms. Drizzle with the
vinaigrette and toss to coat well. Sprinkle with walnuts and serve immediately.

Tips
Make Ahead Tip: Refrigerate the dressing (Step 1) for up to 2 days.
The oil and nuts in this salad provide a heart-healthy balance of omega-6 to omega-3 fats,
a generous amount of antioxidants and a good supply of protein and fiber.
Nutrition Information (per serving)
211
Calories
19g
Fat
10g
Carbs
4g
Protein

Tofu Cucumber Salad with Spicy Peanut Dressing
Prep Time:
25 mins
Additional Time:
30 mins
Total Time:
55 mins
Servings:
4
Yield:
4 servings
Nutrition Profile:
Low-Carb Diabetes-Appropriate Dairy-Free Healthy Pregnancy Low-Sodium Low Added Sugar Heart-Healthy Vegan Vegetarian Egg-Free Low-calorie.
INGREDIENTS
Hot Peanut Dressing
A quarter of a cup of natural peanut butter
One spoonful of soy sauce with lower sodium
One-tspn rice vinegar
1 ½ tsp darkly roasted sesame oil
One teaspoon of garlicky black bean sauce
one tsp finely chopped fresh ginger

1/4 tspn Sriracha or chile-garlic sauce, or to taste1/2 tsp sugar 1/2 tsp freshly chopped
garlic
1/4 teaspoon ground black pepper from Sichuan
Lettuce
Eight ounces Water-packed tofu with additional firmness, drained, and sliced into
1/2-inch chunks
Quarter one big English cucumber and cut into 3/4-inch-thick slices.
¼ cup chopped salty roasted peanuts, divided into one cup of finely chopped cilantro
¼ cup of finely sliced green onions
DIRECTIONS
To make the dressing, place the peanut butter, soy sauce, vinegar, sesame oil, ginger,
chile-garlic sauce (or Sriracha), ground peppercorns, sugar, and garlic in a medium-sized
bowl. Whisk to thoroughly mix the ingredients.
To make the salad, combine 3/4 cup cilantro, cucumber, and tofu in a big bowl. After
adding two tablespoons of the dressing, toss to coat well. After covering, chill for half an
hour.
Move the salad to a serving dish for serving. Pour over the leftover dressing. Add the
peanuts, scallions, and leftover cilantro on top.
Nutrition Information (per serving)
167 Calories
12g Fat, 7g Carbohydrates
10 grams of protein

Simple Vegan Pesto Zoodles
Prep Time:
25 mins
Additional Time:
5 mins
Total Time:
30 mins
Servings:4

1/4 tspn Sriracha or chile-garlic sauce, or to taste1/2 tsp sugar 1/2 tsp freshly chopped
garlic
1/4 teaspoon ground black pepper from Sichuan
Lettuce
Eight ounces Water-packed tofu with additional firmness, drained, and sliced into
1/2-inch chunks
Quarter one big English cucumber and cut into 3/4-inch-thick slices.
¼ cup chopped salty roasted peanuts, divided into one cup of finely chopped cilantro
¼ cup of finely sliced green onions
DIRECTIONS
To make the dressing, place the peanut butter, soy sauce, vinegar, sesame oil, ginger,
chile-garlic sauce (or Sriracha), ground peppercorns, sugar, and garlic in a medium-sized
bowl. Whisk to thoroughly mix the ingredients.
To make the salad, combine 3/4 cup cilantro, cucumber, and tofu in a big bowl. After
adding two tablespoons of the dressing, toss to coat well. After covering, chill for half an
hour.
Move the salad to a serving dish for serving. Pour over the leftover dressing. Add the
peanuts, scallions, and leftover cilantro on top.
Nutrition Information (per serving)
167 Calories
12g Fat, 7g Carbohydrates
10 grams of protein
Simple Vegan Pesto Zoodles
Prep Time:
25 mins
Additional Time:
5 mins
Total Time:
30 mins
Servings:4